For the last ten years, **Jane Matthews** has been a carer again for the third time, gaining an even greater understanding and knowledge of what being a carer involves and the challenges it entails – personal, emotional and practical. She has now been a carer for three elderly relatives – her mum and two uncles – for over twenty (*twenty!*) years. She has come to realise that the most important message she can give her readers is the importance of self-care.

Aside from her caring role, Jane is a writer, accredited coach and facilitator of 'Heal Your Life' workshop programmes. She is the author of a number of self-help books including *Have the Best Year of Your Life*, *Losing a Pet* and *Living Softly* (forthcoming).

Other titles

Communication across Dementia

Challenging Depression and Despair

Free Yourself from Anxiety

Learning to Counsel

Healing the Hurt Within

The Carer's Handbook

Third Edition

Essential Information and Support for
All Those in a Caring Role

Jane Matthews

ROBINSON

ROBINSON

First published in Great Britain in 2006 by
How To Books Ltd

This revised and updated edition published in
Great Britain in 2019 by Robinson

A CIP catalogue record for this book is
available from the British Library

ISBN: 978-1-47214-187-3

Typeset in Sentinel by
Initial Typesetting Services, Edinburgh
Printed and bound in Great Britain
by Clays Ltd, Elcograf S.p.A.

Papers used by Robinson are from well-
managed forests and other responsible
sources

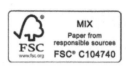

Robinson
An imprint of
Little, Brown Book Group
Carmelite House
50 Victoria Embankment
London EC4Y 0DZ

An Hachette UK Company
www.hachette.co.uk

www.littlebrown.co.uk

....

NOTE: The material contained in this book
is set out in good faith for general guidance
and no liability can be accepted for loss
or expense incurred as a result of relying
in particular circumstances on statements
made in the book. Laws and regulations are
complex and liable to change, and readers
should check the current position with the
relevant authorities before making personal
arrangements.

....

CONTENTS

Introduction: Hello – Good to See You Here ... xiii

Chapter 1 Becoming a Carer 1

Are *you* a carer? **1**

Out of sight, out of mind **2**

Your choice to care **3**

Why recognising you're a carer matters **4**

Living your values is a choice, too **5**

You are not alone **6**

Chapter 2 Finding Your Way through the Care Maze 8

What's stopping you from asking for help? **9**

Understanding who does what **11**

Local government **11**

Health services **12**

Government services **13**

Voluntary services **14**

Chapter 3 **Getting to Grips with Community Care and Financial Assessments** 17

Care Act or needs assessment **18**

What you need to know about community care assessments **19**

Involving the person you're caring for **20**

Assessments for children **21**

The financial assessment **22**

Direct payments **24**

The carer's assessment **26**

Chapter 4 **Working with the Professionals** 29

Being a part of the team **31**

Tips on being a good team player **32**

What to do if you hit a brick wall **33**

A crash course in being assertive **34**

Keeping records **35**

Chapter 5 **Money Matters** 36

Paying for services **36**

Knowing which benefits are available **37**

What could you and your loved one be entitled to? **38**

Other sources of support **40**

To apply or not to apply **41**

Looking after someone else's money **42**

Bank and savings accounts **43**

Lasting Power of Attorney **43**

Making a Will **45**

Practicalities **45**

Difficult conversations **46**

Controlling spending **46**

Chapter 6 More on Money – Help for You As
            a Carer **48**

The high cost of caring **48**

Your pension **50**

Get financially savvy **50**

Tips from carers **51**

Chapter 7 Working through It – Carers and
            the World of Work **53**

A little help from the law **54**

Employers who care **55**

Deciding whether to stay or go **57**

Staying employable **58**

Being a carer is a job, too **59**

Chapter 8 Home Sweet Home **61**

The 'where' of care **62**

The special challenges of caring at a distance **63**

Need to know checklist **66**

Making the environment work for you **67**

Common equipment and adaptations to consider **68**

Getting organised **69**

Staying safe **70**

Creating a good environment for you both **71**

Chapter 9 Staying Healthy as a Carer 73

Carrying out medical procedures 74

Moving and handling 75

Mobility and getting around 76

The taboo of incontinence 78

Self-care 80

High-speed health tips 80

More food for thought 81

Fit for life 82

Mind your mind 83

Chapter 10 Warning: Rocky Relationships Ahead 85

Becoming a parent to your parent 86

Continuing to be child and parent 87

Caring for a partner 89

Let's talk about sex 91

Communication is key 92

Children who remain dependent 93

Returning to the nest 94

Family matters 95

Change your perspective, change your relationships 97

How caring can affect those closest to home 99

Sandwich carers 100

It's not all bad 101

Chapter 11 Some Guidance for Young Carers 103

Get in touch with a carers centre 104

Young carers have rights 105

Getting an assessment **106**

A charter for young carers **106**

Chapter 12 So, How Are You Feeling? 108

Feel those feelings **110**

How to feel, express and release your feelings **111**

Whose life is it anyway? Feelings of loss **112**

Feeling the fury **113**

First aid for dealing with anger **115**

Feelings of resentment **116**

Guilty as charged **117**

All by myself **118**

Anxiety attack **120**

No worries **121**

Should I get help? **122**

Carer's creed **122**

Chapter 13 Survival 123

Understanding depression and despair **124**

How to recognise stress **125**

Setting boundaries **126**

Changing your thinking **128**

Chapter 14 Hundreds of Ways to Get Help 130

Paid carers and care agencies **131**

How will we pay for this care? **132**

How do I know whether it's working? **133**

Day centres and lunch clubs **134**

Holidays and respite **135**

Family and friends **137**

What if my loved one objects? **138**

Other paid help **138**

Chapter 15 Getting Support for You 140

Finding and asking for help **141**

How easy do you find it to ask for help? **142**

Join a carers centre or support group **145**

Get connected **147**

Seek counselling **148**

Phone the family, phone a friend **149**

Help list **150**

Extreme self-care **151**

Chapter 16 Review, Review, Review 153

Stop, look, listen to see what's changed **153**

Recognising when something needs to change **155**

Questions to consider **156**

Chapter 17 Moving to Residential Care 157

Seeing the possibilities in change **158**

Choosing residential care **159**

What to look for and what to ask **160**

Paying for residential care **161**

Continuing to care **163**

Chapter 18 Beyond Caring 165

An end to caring **166**

When the one you are caring for dies **166**

Dealing with the practicalities of death **168**

Riding the emotional roller-coaster **170**

Facing up to the future **172**

Care plan for former carers **174**

Chapter 19 Caring for the Carers 176

Professionals – how to help us help you **177**

Supporting your family member who is a carer **178**

Carers' tips for carers **179**

Resources 181

National Carers Organisations **182**

Other Sources of Information, Advice and Helplines for Carers **182**

Support for Young Carers **184**

Useful Links to Government Services **185**

Sources of Advice on Money, Debt, Benefits, Health and Social Care,
  Rights and Legal Matters **186**

Counselling Services **187**

Grant-making and Practical Support Services **188**

Mental Health Organisations **188**

Work, Education and Training **190**

Home Care, Residential Care and Hospices **191**

Disability and Accessibility **193**

Holidays and Respite **194**

Bereavement **195**

Pets **196**

Information and Support Groups for Specific Conditions **196**

Further Reading **202**

Acknowledgements 205

Index 207

Hello – Good to See You Here . . .

My life as a carer began without me even noticing. My uncle was diagnosed with cancer and I was the only family member living close enough to help. Every weekend I piled my two young children into the car and took him to get his groceries and dry cleaning, and to the fish-and-chip shop for lunch.

A year passed and somehow the shopping trips were the least of it. Little by little I became my uncle's personal assistant, his taxi service and spokesperson. I ferried him to the doctor's and to hospital appointments, paid his bills and made his phone calls. I took his six cats to the vet, arranged for a cleaner and a home meals service. And I kept the rest of our family, geographically far-flung, in touch with his condition.

At home, two lively under-ten-year-olds also wanted my time and attention. And there was the small matter of keeping my job going. The weeks and months flew by – a mad flurry of constant activity – but just about manageable so long as nothing unexpected or extra cropped up.

Inevitably it did. One of the children would be sick or there'd be an impossible deadline at work, or I'd get a late-night phone call from my uncle who was feeling unwell and wanted to be taken to hospital. It ought to have helped, having round-the-clock-care for him in hospital. But the fifty-mile round trip to visit only made life more complicated as I dashed from work to the hospital to his flat where the cats needed feeding, then back in time to collect the children from the childminder's.

I felt like an overwound clock, the cable connecting me to all these commitments ready to snap if anyone exerted the least bit of extra pressure on it. I woke in the early hours and my brain crashed into gear, making endless lists of all the things I needed to do when day finally dawned. Even things that ought to have been a pleasure, like meeting up with friends, became a chore; my heart sank whenever the phone rang. Everything was just another item to add to my 'to do' list.

When ignorance is not bliss

Because of the way I just 'fell' into becoming my uncle's carer, it never occurred to me that I might have any choice in whether to continue. Two hundred miles away, my mother was caring for her two aunts. Looking after family was just something you did if you were needed. My uncle never tired of telling me that the worst thing he could imagine was not being able to continue in his flat, surrounded by his beloved cats. And none of the district nurses who came to change the bandages on his swollen legs, or the hospital staff who summoned me to make arrangements each time he was ready to go home, ever suggested there might be more practical help available for us both.

There were so many things I didn't know.

Reduced hours at work, extra petrol and childcare costs meant money was tight but no one we encountered ever suggested I might be able to claim some financial support for these expenses.

I didn't know about home care assessments, so when we thought that a piece of equipment or minor alteration to the flat might help my uncle with daily life, he paid for it and I organised it.

I didn't know about day centres, or paid carers who might share my load. I didn't know that we were both entitled to a proper home-from-hospital plan each time he was discharged, sicker and weaker, but still determined to stay in his own place. I didn't even know who did what and therefore who I should be talking to about the myriad problems that daily life presented.

Past caring

My caring role lasted five years and, in that time, I never once considered that I might be getting anything out of it. I felt frustration more often than I felt tenderness, and any compassion was tempered by my uncle's apparent lack of awareness of what his sickness was costing me. Having lived alone most of his life he was often argumentative, opinionated and always demanding; only to the hospital and district nurses was he sweetness itself, sending me out to buy them chocolates and flowers.

Eventually, just a few weeks before he died, my uncle's cancer became too advanced for us to manage the pain at home so I moved him into a hospice. He wanted me to stay with him day and night. He was scared of the dark. So I asked work for more time off and spent as many hours as I could sitting by his bed.

This new routine continued until, finally, I collapsed. I came home from a long shift at the hospice and sunk on to the bathroom floor, unable to speak. My children phoned a friend who ordered me to bed and phoned the hospice to say I needed a break for a day or so.

My batteries were totally flat. No longer kept alive by my energy, my uncle let go. He died late the next day.

I believe that it was my friend's act of strength on my behalf, giving me permission to stop, that saved me from breaking down completely. As carers, we seem to find it almost impossible to care for ourselves the way we care for whoever it is we're looking after.

Why I wrote this book

After my uncle's death, I determined to write the guide I wish someone had handed me all those years before when it finally dawned that there was a name for what I was doing.

No two carers face the same situation and yet what we need is remarkably similar: advice on which services are available and how to get hold of them; guidance on finances, home and health; support in dealing with the difficult feelings which add to our load and in handling relationships altered by our caring role. Plus a reminder of what choices we may still have.

Maybe even a tiny bit of recognition.

I wanted the guide to offer carers like you and me all of those things I didn't know I didn't know, so that as long as you choose to go on caring, you have the information and resources you need to hand.

Back to the caring classroom

Since those first two editions of *The Carer's Handbook* appeared, I have become a carer again – this time for the mother I always considered indestructible.

Nine years ago, my endlessly busy, bossy and tough-as-old-boots mum was felled by a stroke. My sister and I cared for her in our own homes for the first six months while we waited to see how much of her speech and movement she'd recover. When it became clear she could no longer manage without support, we boxed up her home on the south coast and sold it in exchange for a tiny cottage next to my sister, where she could be cared for by us and an army of paid carers provided by adult social care.

This time around, of course, I'd literally 'written the book'. So I knew about the practicalities: who I needed to talk to and what I needed to do in order to activate the complex mechanism of official support – doctors, nurses, medical specialists, adult social workers, financial assessors, paid carers, private carers, blue badge assessments, and the tortuous rigmarole of form-filling that government requires.

It turned out, though, that there was another important element to being a carer that I had yet to learn: how to care properly and committedly for myself.

You see, even though my sister and I both knew we needed sometimes to put ourselves first if we were to have the resources to continue caring, in the face of Mum's increasing frailty and dependence on us, we found it so easy to ignore our own needs.

Three years ago, my sister had a breakdown, forcing her to give up work entirely for six months. Then, late last year, unable to think of a single reason to get out of bed, I recognised that I'd also reached burnout. The positive thing about burnout is that it forces you to stop and review what you believe and how you are living your life. It was salutary for me to realise that no matter how many times I advised others to take care of themselves, it had been a case of 'do what I say, not what I do'.

So I came back to this book, knowing I wanted to beef up the sections that focus on keeping you, the carer, healthy, happy and sane – so you can go on being the best carer you can be for as long as you choose to go on caring.

Who cares?

You see, if *you* don't care for you, who will?

Try as they might, it won't be the health services, the doctors and nurses and hospitals who often fail to spot that behind every person who is sick or living with a disability, or simply growing old, there is usually someone caring for them, whether or not they label themselves 'carer'. Neither will it be the confusion of social and benefits services which make up our welfare state, so often too starved of funds and time to join the dots seamlessly and spot the millions of families, friends, partners and neighbours getting on with the job, who desperately need support.

So who cares for the carer?

I'm afraid it *has* to be us . . .

So that's the spirit in which this new edition is written, as a source of practical information, advice and other carers' experiences to help you on your way. As an act of friendship and support for all of you who will recognise elements of my story in your own lives. And as a reminder that surviving life as a carer means, above all, being your own carer, too.

A few thoughts on using this book

It was important for me to recognise that mine is only one experience of caring; other people do it differently for different reasons and have different experiences, so I wanted to include as many other carers' voices in this book as I could. Sometimes, just hearing from other carers, or sharing my own stories, made a world of difference to how I was feeling. I hope the same will be true for you.

One of the things some of them said was that they had never really found the right term to describe the person they care for. I hugely admire Hugh Marriott's decision to coin the expression 'piglet' (person I give love and endless therapy to) for his book *The Selfish Pig's Guide to Caring*. But in the end, the term that sits best with me is 'loved one'.

So many carers I interviewed said that the bottom line for them was the love they felt for the person they were caring for. That's why they did it, even though there were days and months and even years when that love was buried beneath a slurry heap of other emotions.

That won't be true for everyone reading this book – our relationships are often more messy and complicated than that. So if the 'loved one' phrase doesn't sit well with you then please feel free to substitute 'piglet' or 'person I care for' or any other expression that suits you better. And, by the way, you have no idea how much I admire you for stepping up as a carer when your feelings for the person you are supporting *are* so much more complex.

Finally, you may find it helpful to skim read the whole book first to see what is here and which sections are most useful to you at whatever stage on the caring journey you have reached. One of the things about being a carer is that it involves juggling so many balls at one time. The chapters ahead reflect that, with a huge amount to know, to think about, and to practise. I don't want you to feel overwhelmed, which is why I suggest you may want to take an overview first on what's in the book, before returning to look at the detail of the chapters that will support you the most right now.

CHAPTER 1

Becoming a Carer

'I wish I'd realised I was a carer earlier. By the time the penny dropped, I'd been doing it for decades without any self-awareness or self-care. If I'd known earlier, I would have sought out counselling and understood I needed to have a sympathetic ear to vent my frustrations to.'

Michele

Are *you* a carer?

All her life, Connie was a carer but she'd never have described herself in that way. When she nursed two husbands through terminal illness, she was simply being a wife. Bringing up a daughter with a severe learning disability until she was ready to move into supported accommodation, Connie was just doing what any mother would. As for all the other visits that filled her days? That's what neighbours do for each other.

Right now it's estimated that there are some seven million people in the UK who could be described as carers. But nobody really knows, because of all those like Michele and Connie; they're busy getting on with it without ever knowing that there is a word to describe what they're doing and, therefore, that there are services to support them.

If your child has special needs, if you are doing a relative's shopping or gardening, if your partner suffers periods of depression that they wouldn't survive without your support, if your parent is in residential care and it's you who visits three times a week and liaises with the staff, if your single mum can't cope on her own and you're helping bring up your brothers and sisters, then you're a carer.

Carers Trust says 'a carer is anyone who cares, unpaid, for a friend or family member who due to illness, disability, a mental health problem or an addiction cannot cope without their support'. It doesn't matter whether you're spending a few hours a week taking someone to their medical appointments or you're looking after someone round-the-clock, 365 days a year. If you're not being paid then you're a carer.

Out of sight, out of mind

It's because every carer's situation is so different that we may find it hard to recognise ourselves. It's so easy to think of other people who are having a harder time, who are having to do a great deal more than we do.

Carers I've interviewed for this book almost always qualify any woes or complaints by assuring me they know other people have it much harder. I felt the same when I was telling you about my caring roles in the Introduction. OK, it's been almost two decades but at least I've always been able to escape back behind my own front door. At least I've been able to continue doing some paid work. I haven't had to give up my friendships. Carers are people forced to give up everything to look after someone else, aren't they?

The other thing that may stop us recognising ourselves as carers is living in a society for whom we are often invisible – despite the fact that, according to Carers Trust, *three in five of us will be carers at some point in our lives in the UK*. Just consider:

- Have you ever been given the chance to tick a box labelled *'and carer'* on a form that asks for your occupation?
- At the library or bookstore, have you ever spotted a section for carers similar to those for gardening or cooking or any other occupation seven million people are involved in?
- When you chat to friends or colleagues, how able do you feel to share the details of what being a carer involves for you?
- How often when you are talking to health or social services about the person you're caring for do they ask, 'And how are you?'
- Has any part of officialdom stepped in to offer to fully reimburse you for the lost working hours, or the additional outgoings on everything from travel to laundry to food on the go?

'As every carer knows, to become a carer is to become invisible. Invisible, helpless and, all too often, hopeless. How can this be? How can even our most minor "celebrity" command more column inches in our newspapers than this army of people who – unpaid and unlauded – are doing one of the most important jobs a person can do?'

Marianne Talbot in *Keeping Mum: Caring for Someone with Dementia*

Your choice to care

Another reason we may not notice we're signed-up members of this invisible army of carers is because of the way so many of us simply fall into it, as I did with my uncle.

For Graeme, there was no single moment when life turned upside down. It was just that his widowed father seemed to need more and more from him. 'I didn't wake up one morning and think that's it – I'll be his carer. But when I met up with friends, I'd realise that I didn't have much to talk about apart from looking after Dad. Apart from getting up and going to work, that was all I did. There wasn't time for anything else.'

'You don't choose it. It chooses you,' is how Stephanie puts it. She gave up a teaching career to nurse her partner when he was paralysed from the neck down in a road accident. 'It was never a question of choice. The hospital said Gerry wouldn't walk so I just got on and fixed things at home so I could take over.'

Many of us would agree that we didn't actively choose to be carers. Like Graeme and Stephanie, it's something life thrust on us. Something we do out of love for the person we're caring for, out of a sense of duty or responsibility – or because we think no one else will. In every life, things happen and we do our best to cope.

How did *you* get here? Do you feel as if you had a choice?

Why recognising you're a carer matters

The thing is, recognising you're a carer and recognising that every day you go on caring you are – at some level – choosing to go on doing so *really* matters. Maybe not to the part of our world for whom we are invisible, but to ourselves – our mental and physical well-being and sense of ourselves.

Here's why.

Supporting someone else to have the best quality of life they can is one of the most life-affirming things we can do with *our* time. From those who are dying, we hear this truth repeatedly: that when our time comes, what will count is not the hours we spent in the office or chasing the things society told us we should want, but the time we spent on human connection, with family and friends, loving and being loved.

That's the positive side of being a carer. The challenging side is that caring can sometimes be stressful, demanding, emotional and lonely.

Whatever your circumstances, the moment the 'Oh, I'm a carer' light goes on over your head is the moment you can start thinking about the ways in which you need to start caring for yourself, too. You start to have choices about accessing the help and support that exists out there for you.

Someone once told me that becoming a carer is a bit like crossing a road without a kerb. Normally, the kerb is our signal to stop, pay attention and look around for the sake of our safety. When there's no kerb, it's hard to say where the journey begins. We are underway before we realise it, suddenly aware of cars hurtling towards us.

Let me say that again, because if you take nothing else from this book and the experiences of every carer I have ever spoken to, it is this: *you have to care for yourself. You matter as much as your loved one and your ability to go on caring for them depends on you knowing that and acting on it. If you don't, then one of those cars is going to hit you.*

Living your values is a choice, too

Moving home can be one of the most stressful experiences we can put ourselves through as we wait on other people, contracts, dead-slow solicitors, and systems belonging to the Dark Ages. The stresses of caring are remarkably similar, above all the sense that events are out of our control. Events that affect our lives profoundly depend entirely on the actions and choices of others. We feel stress most acutely when we believe we have no control or choice over our own lives.

As you allow yourself to recognise you are a carer then thinking about how you got here and why you do what you do may help you to take back a little of that control. When we say we have no choice we are forgetting who we are, forgetting that acting on the compassion we feel, honouring our belief in the importance of family, friendship, neighbourliness, even duty, are very much choices.

These are your values; the qualities that make you *you*. If tomorrow you wake up and decide you don't want to be a carer any longer, then someone else will have to pick up the pieces, however imperfect, inconvenient or inadequate that might be. Each day you wake up and continue with the business of being a carer – no matter the size or shape of your commitment, whether you do it in their home, remotely or in a residential home, for one hour or thousands – you are choosing to live your values.

And, by the way, you are also making the world a fractionally better, kinder place for all of us.

> *'Mum and I had a massive row and in the middle of it she shouted, "Why are you doing this anyway?" It stopped me in my tracks; we didn't have the kind of relationship where we spoke about serious stuff. I mumbled something about wanting to help her, helping her stay in her home, about knowing she'd do the same for me. She didn't say anything for a while but she was shaking her head. "You do it because we love each other," she said and I realised she was right. That was what it was about.'*
>
> Maureen

You Are Not Alone

Carers tell me that it's one of the loneliest jobs there is – which is ironic when you see how many of us there are:

- Around 7 million people in the UK are carers – one in ten of us is looking after ill, disabled or elderly partners, children, relatives, friends and neighbours.

- By 2030 that figure will rise to around 10.4 million (or one in seven of us) as our population lives longer.
- 42 per cent of UK carers are men and 58 per cent are women.
- A survey by the BBC in 2010 estimated there are around 700,000 'young (school-age) carers' in the UK.
- At the other end of the scale, one in five people aged 50–64 are carers.
- Also on the rise are 'sandwich carers' – according to a YouGov poll in 2012, 2.4 million people carry the dual responsibility of caring for young children alongside elderly or disabled relatives.

Figures: Carers Trust 2018

CHAPTER 2

Finding Your Way through the Care Maze

'Dad had been in the nursing home for nine months before I stumbled on a reference to Continuing Nursing Care – it was in a magazine article. The article said some people in care homes can qualify for a contribution from the health authority towards their fees. Well, after a long assessment process we heard he not only qualified, they'd pay his nursing home fees in full. But what if I'd never read that magazine?'

Julie

For most things in life, there's a recognised 'gateway' you can go to to get help and information from experts. If you're moving house you visit an estate agent who'll guide you through the process. If you want to book a holiday, the travel agent will take the strain (and your money).

Caring's not like that. Instead of a one-stop shop, you're confronted with a row of doors leading to a maze of arcades; and instead of joining up, each arcade leads only to a whole row of more doors – and sometimes dead ends.

I'd been caring for years before one particularly lovely adult social worker heard the wobble in my voice and suggested I should get a carer's assessment. Because carrying it out was contracted out to the local carers support group, that then became a gateway to proper tea, sympathy and all the vast array of resources that carer support organisations hold.

But why did it take so long? Why did the 2017 'State of Caring' report from Carers UK find that although two-thirds of carers say their doctors know about their caring role, they don't offer any extra support as a result? Or why did a survey reported in Carers Trust's 'Key Facts about Carers' find that 35 per cent of carers are missing out on state benefits because they didn't realise they could claim them?

That's an awful lot of people passing under the radar of health and social services, considering that, together, those services form the gateway to a whole range of support.

So that's the first problem: discovering what it is you don't know.

In this chapter, I want to give an overview of the kinds of support that might be available and who provides them. I've also included a general checklist at the end of the chapter so you don't have to try and remember everything you read.

What's stopping you from asking for help?

But before we go there, I want to make the case for taking a deep breath and tackling the care maze. It's tempting, I know, the first time you are confronted with the twenty tightly packed pages of a financial assessment or blue badge application form to hurl them through the window and swear you'll damn well go it alone.

There's the time factor; you've already got your hands full being a carer. How on earth are you expected to conjure up non-existent time for appointments and meetings, form-filling and telephone calls?

Or perhaps you fear that bringing in outside agencies will mean giving up what little control you have. You think the moment health or social services poke their heads round the door they'll make the rules and life will become even more complicated than it already is.

Alternatively, you may – like so many of us – be suffering from that well-known carers' complaint – the curse of the strong. Like Tony who told me how close he came to breaking under the strain of caring for his severely disabled wife and their daughter with Downs Syndrome: 'Being a male carer, I was seen by everyone as being in charge, as coping, while inside I was screaming. I wasn't good at asking for help – but if I had asked, I would have seen that as me failing. It was up to me to look after them.'

We're copers – until the day we're not.

And that's the thing. Ten years on, Tony says if he had his time again he'd do it differently: 'Tell people not to do what I did. As carers, we have to preserve ourselves. All the time I was getting on with it alone I neglected my own needs.'

Those agencies that do offer some support to carers say it's often only when people reach crisis point that they hear from them. But just think how much harder it is to do anything when you're in crisis – you're feeling emotional, not thinking straight and you're desperate for something to change *now*.

I won't try to kid you that getting involved in the care maze isn't complicated, time-consuming and often downright infuriating. But the clue is in the name – our government, health, social and voluntary *services* exist to *serve*. It's their job to put you in touch with the practical, medical and financial support that will make life a little easier for you and the person you care for. They'll also be your back-up should a crisis arise.

Understanding who does what

There are four sectors you may want or need to deal with:

- Local government – the local council where you and the person you're caring for live (and possibly two councils if you live in different areas). They're primarily responsible for the practicalities of providing care as part of daily life.
- Health services – GP surgeries, hospitals and a whole raft of specialists for everything from incontinence to end-of-life care.
- Central government – I'm talking mainly about our benefits system and financial support for you and your loved one.
- Voluntary services – the charities and support groups, including those specifically for carers, that pick up so many of the pieces.

From here on, when I'm talking about the people whose job is to support you, I shall call them the 'professionals'. That's not because you're not a professional – most unpaid carers I've met do a better job than even the most committed professional who is paid to care. I just want to save you ploughing through more words than you need to.

Details of who does what, and who you're most likely to come across, are spelt out below.

Local government

Social worker – Social services departments at your local council are where you will find social workers, who may be called 'case workers' or 'care managers'. They're responsible for the assessments of the person you care for – and for you as their carer, for producing the 'care plan', and also for liaising with other areas of the local council's services that may need to be involved, such as day centres, home care, education services and child health.

Financial assessor – Council care plans come at a cost for which your loved one may be liable, depending on their income. Once the care plan is agreed, the council will arrange for a financial assessor to work out what, if any, contribution they require.

Care assistants – Care assistants support people to stay in their own homes and to provide cover for you, the carer. For instance, they may help with getting your loved one into and out of bed, washing, dressing, going to the toilet and with household tasks such as cooking and shopping.

Other social services – These may include support services such as night sitting, and care facilities outside the home such as day centres, residential homes and respite care. Again, the social worker and care plan are the starting points for these services.

Health services

Doctor or GP – Your first point of contact for getting general medical advice, and for referring you on to specialists and involving other health services such as district nurses.

As soon as you can, get your loved one's permission for you to speak to their doctor on their behalf and ensure it's noted on their records. And make sure you tell your own doctor you're a carer so your own health doesn't get overlooked.

District nurse – The doctor will call in the district nurse if the person you're caring for has nursing needs which are best carried out at home; for instance, changing dressings or giving injections.

Community psychiatric or mental health nurse – The community psychiatric nurse supports people with mental health problems, and those around them, by providing advice, administering medication and keeping an eye on the way the patient is doing under any care and treatment they receive.

Other specialists – There is an army of health professionals who may be called in to help your loved one with the specifics or symptoms of their condition or disability. These include: speech therapist, continence adviser, dietician, low vision specialist, physiotherapist and occupational therapist. They will all advise on adaptations, equipment and practical aids in the home. If you think any of these services would be useful, and no one has suggested them, talk to the doctor or social worker.

Hospital – As part of their illness or disability, the person you're caring for may need hospital treatment or be referred to medical specialists based at the local hospital. Be aware that the hospital will keep an entirely different set of records from the doctor's surgery and that letters of referral are unlikely to contain much more than the bare facts, so be prepared to tell the whole story again!

Home-from-hospital co-ordinator – If your loved one has been hospitalised, they shouldn't be sent home until the co-ordinator has produced a new care plan and contacted all the professionals who are involved in delivering it. Depending on their condition, that could include up to six weeks' free rehabilitation support.

Hospice – Hospices are experts in the care of people with terminal or degenerative conditions and, although most are run as charities, referrals are usually via the health service. Many hospices also run day centres and offer respite care.

Government services

I've included these in the list because, although you'll usually be dealing with a system rather than named individuals, there is a growing amount of advice for carers on the Government website www.gov.uk. The resources section at the back of this book will signpost you to some of the areas of this vast website that are likely to be most useful to you for information on benefits, allowances, pensions and more.

Voluntary services

From Macmillan and Marie Curie providing expert support for cancer patients, through Age UK's excellent raft of services, we'd be lost without our brilliant voluntary sector. There are too many to include in this short list so the names below are only a starting point; you'll find more suggestions in the resources section.

Carers centres – Let's start with two giants I've already mentioned: Carers Trust (https://carers.org) and Carers UK (www.carersuk.org). Both offer comprehensive, clear and up-to-date information for carers everywhere. Carers Trust also supports carers where they live through a UK network of independent carers centres. There are around 150 of these, offering a wide range of services, from assistance with the carer's assessment and claiming benefits through to accessing education and training. They also offer the relief of being heard by people who understand what it means to be a carer.

Age UK – Not every carer is looking after someone elderly or in mid-life themselves. But for those who are, Age UK is a goldmine of clearly set out information on many of the issues you're likely to come across. Around 150 local branches also offer practical support services such as befriending, home help, handyperson, gardening, footcare and more.

British Red Cross – This well-known charity can loan medical equipment such as wheelchairs, and may assist with care in the home, transport needs and first-aid training.

Citizens Advice – This is an excellent source of free information and advice on all kinds of things, but especially in making sense of benefits and bureaucracy. Their trained volunteers can help you complete some of those scary forms.

Specialist support groups – Whatever the reason the child or adult you are caring for needs help, from a rare genetic condition to simple old age, there will be a support group set up by and for people going through the same experience as both of you. These groups are absolute experts at what they do. They've been on the front line and they know what works and what doesn't. Talk to them. Lean on them. Use them.

Here's a checklist of ten things to consider when you recognise you're a carer:

1. Even if you've become a carer because your loved one has had a health crisis, try not to rush in with guns blazing. It's so tempting to take on the world but, believe me, it's so much harder to disengage once you've committed yourself. Crisis or no, you need to stop, draw breath and make time to deal with both the practical and emotional implications for your life.

2. Call a family meeting to talk through what's happening, what may happen, what are the care options now and into the future, and who is going to be responsible for what. (It won't necessarily be plain sailing; see Chapter 10 on relationships.)

3. Contact adult social services at your local council and ask for a care assessment for your loved one and carer's assessment for you. (Even if you think things aren't yet 'bad or difficult enough', these assessments will set a baseline and make unlocking services in future a little quicker: see Chapter 3.)

4. Buy a notebook – dates, phone numbers, conversations, diagnoses will take on an inordinate importance once you enter the care maze so it's never too soon to start writing things down. (See Chapter 4 on working with the professionals.)

5. Get some idea of what benefits you and/or they might be entitled to; contact one of the helplines run by carers centres, the Citizens Advice or Age UK. Use one of the online benefit check tools: www.entitledto.co.uk or www.turn2us.org.uk, and read Chapter 5.

6. If you think the person you're caring for is likely to get worse rather than better, then help them set in train a Lasting Power of Attorney application. There are two types: for financial matters and for health and care matters. (See Chapter 3 on health and Chapter 5 on money matters.)

7. If you're working, let your employer know your circumstances have changed. (You have some legal rights but it also makes sense to have your employer on side – see Chapter 7.)

8. Let your doctor know you've become a carer and let your loved one's doctor know you are caring for their patient so you've permission to help with medical affairs. (There's advice on all things health in Chapter 9.)

9. Do a mental audit of your own support systems. Do you have enough? Are they giving you the resilience you need as a carer? (If you haven't already realised that I think supporting *you* is vital, then re-read the Introduction and see Chapter 15.)

10. Have a long, hard think about the things that make your life worth living and commit to continuing to make time for at least some of them. (And while you're at it, take a look at Chapter 12 – how you feel matters.)

CHAPTER 3

Getting to Grips with Community Care and Financial Assessments

As I pointed out at the end of the last chapter, one of the keys to getting support for you and your loved one is to get assessed.

There are three separate assessments you need to know about:

- The Care Act assessment – at which social services will carry out a thorough review of your loved one's needs and abilities and determine how best they can be supported.
- The financial assessment – to determine how much this support is going to cost and how much your loved one will have to contribute towards the costs.
- The carer's assessment – at which they'll look at your situation and support needs.

Because I am mainly writing this book to support you, I'm tempted to start with the carer's assessment. But the reality is it is unlikely to happen in that order, so let's begin where you will almost certainly start.

Care Act or needs assessment

Any adult over eighteen who may need help with daily living is legally entitled to an assessment from the adult social care team. Similarly, if you are caring for a child with special needs, they are entitled to an assessment from children's services.

You don't need a professional referral to ask for this. You or your loved one can trigger the assessment by contacting the relevant team at your local council. A social worker will arrange to visit and go through a long list of the tasks and occupations that are a normal part of everyday life for most of us, for example:

- Are they able to manage their own finances, pay the bills when they're due, budget appropriately?
- Do they need help with any routine day-to-day tasks – preparing and cleaning up after meals, taking tablets, changing dressings or other medical care, getting up, keeping clean, using the toilet, getting dressed or going to bed?
- Are they coping looking after their home, keeping it clean and tidy, managing a garden, looking after pets, keeping the house at the right temperature? Can they do their own laundry?
- Can they occupy themselves, pursue hobbies and interests, and can they get around outside the home – visit friends, do their own shopping, and so on?
- Are there any practical aids or equipment that would make a difference to their ability to stay in their (or your) home and have a reasonable quality of life, such as stairlift, ramps, handrails, alarm system?
- What about adaptations to wherever the caring is taking place; for instance, moving a bedroom downstairs, installing a wet room, lowering units or widening doors?

Those are just a few of the many things that go on day to day that may no longer be running smoothly. But the assessment isn't only about the practicalities but also what's important to your loved one; how they want to spend their time, how they want to be cared for, their priorities as well as their needs.

What you need to know about community care assessments

Everything you discuss at the assessment will be set out in the care plan, which is produced by the social worker and shared with you so you and your loved one can agree it.

Local and national carers centres, which I've already mentioned, provide detailed information about what happens at the assessment, how the council decides whether your loved one is eligible for support, and how this will be delivered. So do speak to them, request a booklet, or check out their online resources, before the assessment. At the same time, let me share a few headlines I hope will be useful:

- Under the terms of the Care Act, your loved one has the right to an advocate, someone to support them or speak on their behalf at the assessment. This could be you, but you might also choose to bring in someone who knows their way around the system, such as an independent social worker, or adviser from a carers centre or support group.
- Use the checklist above to think about how your loved one is coping, where they're not, and what they want and need, before the assessment. If you're able to discuss this together that's ideal, and making notes of what you agree will be invaluable once you are face-to-face with a clipboard and a barrage of questions.
- It's helpful if you have already given some thought to what support would help them – and you. There are many suggestions throughout this book; for instance, paid carers coming in to assist, spells at a day centre for company, or respite care for you.
- Take as much time as you need. It's OK to say you don't know something, and do ask the assessor to explain anything you don't

understand. There's a lot of jargon around social care that can be confusing.

- You don't have to sign the care plan until you're happy with it. Don't be afraid to come back on anything that's been missed, or even changed while the plan was being written.

- On which note, remember that the plan may need to be reviewed at intervals. If your loved one's needs are temporary – for instance, they've just come out of hospital and simply need time to recover – that's good news. But for many, especially elderly people or anyone with a life-limiting illness, the pattern is one of decline – and things that were set up may no longer keep your loved one safe, or maintain their quality of life, after a while.

- Even if you are currently meeting all your loved one's needs, asking for an assessment establishes a baseline that may be helpful if those needs increase; it gets you and them known to social services, and means you have somewhere to turn should a crisis arise.

Involving the person you're caring for

Unless their condition prevents them from having any meaningful role in planning their own care – if they're suffering from dementia for instance – the professionals will want to talk to the person you're caring for and involve them as much as possible in making decisions.

At a time when their disability, illness or condition may have robbed them of their independence, it's important they are not further disempowered by feeling that they're being sidelined or treated as a child.

If you have a good, open relationship and are able to be fairly honest with each other, it probably hasn't occurred to you *not* to involve them in the arrangements that are being made. That way, there should be no uncomfortable surprises for either of you. You may even find they're able to suggest things you haven't thought of. Perhaps they've been longing to pursue a hobby or have friends round or take baths instead of showers, but didn't like to mention it because they're sensitive to how much you are already doing.

Not all relationships are open, however. In even the best relationships, we sometimes stop ourselves from being honest because we're sensitive to hurting those we care about; for instance, by publicly contradicting them every time they insist they can do for themselves the tasks that we're performing.

And then there are relationships where we don't feel we can be honest at all. Life's already hard enough without having to face the consequences of admitting to the social worker in front of your father that the hardest aspect of being his carer is the way he moans incessantly about every single thing you do and say.

If the person you're caring for has come up through the school of stiff upper lips and is uncomfortable talking about anything personal, if they are struggling with being seen as needy or dependent, or don't accept or understand that they are ill, then honesty with each other – and in front of a social worker – may be neither possible nor wise.

What you need to do is ask that the assessment includes time for you and the social worker to talk separately, as well as with the person you're caring for. That way you're in a position to challenge any misapprehensions and ensure the assessor goes away with a truly accurate picture of what is going on.

Assessments for children

For parents caring for children with special needs, much of the same information applies. 'Special needs' means any physical or mental health illness or impairment that is affecting your child's development or quality of life, and that they and you need support with.

The assessment is usually carried out by a social worker in your own home but, depending on your child's age, other services might be involved such as health and education.

Again, the assessment will cover all the help that your disabled child needs but, in addition, unlike adult assessments, the needs of any other children in the family and the help you may need to care for your disabled child will be taken into account.

If no one has suggested an assessment then you can request it yourself by contacting social services, or asking your doctor or any support organisation you're involved with to do it for you. Be clear that you are requesting a Care Act assessment – you have a right to this.

It certainly helps to prepare. Among the things you might want to think about and note down are:

- The impact your child's needs have on their daily life.
- How you and any other family members are affected.
- Any areas where you and they are particularly struggling.
- Their medical history and any involvement to date from health and other support services.
- The sorts of help and support in every area – practical, health care, social, educational and emotional – that might make a difference to you all. For instance:
  - home help, personal care, a sitting service, equipment or adaptations;
  - services outside the home, such as an after-school club or holiday play scheme;
  - help with travel and other social care assistance to enable your child to take part in recreational activities or education;
  - holidays or temporary short breaks or respite care or the provision of accommodation on a longer-term basis.

The financial assessment

The financial assessment is made to determine how much the support in the care plan is going to cost and how much your loved one will have to contribute towards those costs – unless they are a child in which case most services should be free.

How much they are asked to contribute will depend on how much they have in savings and other income. The law on income and savings thresholds is very much up for discussion at the moment and the financial assessor will be able to tell you what those thresholds currently are.

Moreover, what's available varies from area to area according to individual budgets and how needs are assessed. You may end up with a fantastic care plan and then learn that your loved one will have to fund it all.

Do remember, it *is* the person you care for who is expected to pay for services or top-ups, not their partner if they have one, and not you, their carer. But real life is often not as neat as the professionals would like it to be, so we'll be looking in detail at the financial impacts of caring and what you can do about them in later chapters.

Another complication is that some of you will be caring for people brought up to believe there are few greater sins than discussing money in public.

You'll usually be sent a form in advance – and if you aren't, then ask for it because many of the questions involve a lot of research – before an assessor from the council visits to go through the detail with you.

One or both of you will need to have a handle on their income from pensions, investments, benefits they may already be getting as well as the extent of their savings, and other assets such as property – although the value of their home is not currently included in the assessment if they, their partner or, indeed, you are living in it.

It's also vital to be able to show what their existing outgoings are – mortgage or rent, utilities, etc. – and also any expenses that relate directly to their disability, illness or condition – for example, an alarm system, or if you or they are spending a fortune on laundry because they keep having 'accidents'.

However much information you take with you, it's always the crucial bit that seems to be missing, so err on the side of collecting together too much information rather than too little. You don't want to have to go through this process twice.

Direct payments

Let's assume your loved one is on a low income with few savings and, having done their care assessment and financial assessment, social services will be picking up the tab for the home or day care that has been set out in the final care plan.

At this point, you and your loved one have a choice about how this money is spent. One option is to ask social services to manage the budget for you. This doesn't mean you don't still have choices – for instance, which care agency you'd like them to use to provide carers for your loved one. It does mean, though, that all the invoicing and administration is done by them.

The alternative is to request a direct payment which you then use to buy the agreed services and support.

I'll be honest, I held back from writing about this because this will certainly involve you having to keep additional records and, as the Government's own website warns with a large exclamation mark, if you are paying someone to care for your loved one, this could involve you or them becoming an employer.

On the other hand, as carers who have gone down this route tell me, it can give you much greater choice and control over every aspect of how care is provided. So it is worth your time to consider whether the additional work would be outweighed by the benefits to you both.

Before you make a decision, these are the things you might want to consider:

- It is possible to request a mixed package of care, with social services managing some elements of the budget and others coming direct to you or your loved one to spend on their needs?
- If your loved one does not have mental capacity, or does but would be unable to manage a direct payment, you or someone else can be appointed to do it on their behalf – giving you more control, or an opportunity to enlist another family member to help in a practical way.
- It may be possible to use the direct payment to employ you or another family member to look after your loved one.
- The direct payment can only be spent on meeting needs that were agreed in the care plan.
- If you decide to use the money to employ a care worker or workers yourself, then there will be extra costs on top of the salary; for instance, recruitment, national insurance, pension and income tax. The direct payment must cover these as well.
- As more councils and individuals go down the direct payments route there are now organisations in many areas that can help you with employing a care worker directly. These can take on much of the administration for you, so do ask social services if there is a local direct payments support service.
- You can avoid becoming an employer altogether by using a care agency who will then be the employers.
- If you opt for a direct payment you will be required to keep records and send your accounts to the local council to show how the money is being spent.

The carer's assessment

So finally – and with apologies for doing the very thing I have urged you not to do, which is put you last – we come to the carer's assessment.

If you are over eighteen and caring for another adult who is ill, disabled or needs support because of their age, then you're entitled to an assessment of the role's impact on your life and what you need to support you in fulfilling this role. It doesn't matter how much or 'little' (in your view) caring you do; and it doesn't matter whether your loved one is already known to social and health services. If being a carer is having an impact on your life, then it's worth making the time for this. You would be surprised how many different support services it could unlock for you; for example, I've heard of carers being given funds to have a weekly massage, pay for driving lessons or take a break.

If one of the professionals hasn't already suggested this and referred you, then pick up the phone to social services and request it yourself.

You should be sent information in advance to help you think about what you are doing, and how it is affecting everything from your working life through your family life to your social life, relationships, finances, health and emotional well-being.

The following checklist is a starting point. Along with thinking about these things, you could talk to your family and friends about how they perceive what you do, what you need, and how you are being affected. Or keep a diary for a week and note down not only what you're doing for your loved one, but also how much time is involved and how you feel from day to day.

Checklist for preparing for the carer's assessment:

● Note down the tasks you help with: housework, cooking, gardening, laundry, personal care, finances, transport, socialising – to name just a few.

- How many hours does this involve and are these every day, at night time, daily or occasional? Are you 'on call' for your loved one, and having to drop everything to respond when they call?
- Does anyone else help and are there support services in place? What are the areas of providing care where you are struggling and not sure you can continue to cope?
- Are you able to spend enough time on your other responsibilities; for instance, partners, children or other relatives?
- If you are in employment, how is your working life affected? What support do you need to carry on working?
- Do you have any health problems of your own, or is your health being affected by your caring role? For example, are you experiencing stress or is your sleep or diet or even ability to exercise affected?
- How are you feeling day to day? Do you feel you're coping or are there times when you are emotional and feel close to breaking? Is it your choice to continue caring?
- Are there things you love doing that you can't manage any more because of your caring responsibilities?

Let me just add one more thing to the list of what you need to think about: *when you get your assessment, please tell it like it is.* If you're a carer, you're almost certainly trying to be a coper. Copers are wonderful people because they make life so much easier for the rest of us; you say you're OK so we don't need to worry about you or help you out. The social worker is trying to assess your needs and asks, 'How are you?' and you fix a smile on your face and say, 'I'm fine, really.'

Expecting other people to read between the lines is usually a frustrating experience, especially if they themselves are hard pressed and ever conscious of their department's limited budgets.

Don't forget, health and social services need you to do this job.

If you don't, they'll have to, and that's going to be infinitely more complicated and gobble up an awful lot more resources than it will to support you doing the job of carer. So be honest with them.

CHAPTER 4

Working with the Professionals

'The paramedics and the doctors in Accident and Emergency assumed Mum was having a heart attack. It wasn't until I got there and told them she'd had a DVT and a stroke they did a scan and found she had pulmonary embolisms.'

Martha

Formal assessments are likely to be only two or three of many encounters you'll have with those working in the 'paid' caring professions. As well as the health and social care professionals we've already looked at you may need to contact their colleagues in housing, education, employment or the benefits offices.

For you, the needs of the person you're caring for are paramount. For the professionals, no matter how experienced, how good at their job, how committed they are to their clients, you'll be one file in a huge pile on a desk groaning with work.

In order to make the most of the contacts you have with these people who can support you, there are some things you need to keep in mind. The things you need to know about the 'professionals' include:

- *They're not always great at sharing information with each other* – just because you've talked to the case worker, don't expect the home-care assistant to know all about your situation and what's expected of them.
- *They are often too busy to do much more than answer the questions you ask* – before any meeting or appointment, draw up your own list of the things you need to know about. At the end, put them on the spot: 'Is there anything else you think I should know or you need to tell me?'
- *Even in their own records they usually only look at the top page* – what would you do when faced with a file as fat as a brick and only ten minutes scheduled for each appointment? This is especially true of GPs and hospital staff. Never assume when you're talking that they have the whole picture. Be prepared to give a swift potted medical history on every occasion.
- *Unlike you, they usually don't work weekends* – there is an out-of-hours on-call system so you won't be left high and dry. But the person on call may not know you or the person you care for so there may be some scene-setting to do. Do ask your contacts in health and social services to give you names and numbers for emergencies when they can't be reached. And don't leave anything to a Friday if you can help it.
- *It's the person you're caring for who is their priority, not you* – you may not be comfortable putting yourself forward but you do need to remind them that you are your loved one's partner in this caring relationship. Your knowledge and insights count. So do your needs; if they're not being looked after then you won't be in a position to look after anyone else.
- *Mistakes happen when people are stretched and stressed* – if you think they've got something wrong, don't be afraid to say so. We all make mistakes and so will they from time to time. (So will you for that matter.)
- *People talk about 'the system' but there isn't one, so don't expect*

things to happen systematically. As Hugh Marriott points out in his excellent book *The Selfish Pig's Guide to Caring,* the fact that you'll encounter all of the situations above is not a conspiracy to make your life impossible. It's just chaos! A good social worker should be able to help you navigate this.

Being a part of the team

Though there may be days when you feel ignored or invisible, it's vital to keep reminding yourself that, far from being on the sidelines, you are at the very core of a care team. And as part of that team, you are owed the same respect and support as everyone else in it, even if, unlike them, you are not being paid for the work that you do.

You may encounter some professionals who do not always see it that way or who you feel don't listen properly to you or share information. They will, of course, be mindful of client confidentiality but it won't hurt to gently remind them that as your loved one's main carer you are often in the best position to know what will help most.

If you're able, work hard at your relationships with the other members of the team. It may not be fair but it is a fact that the better you and the person you care for are known to them, the more you project yourself as part of a partnership, the more assistance you will both get. Think back to the school classroom and how quickly the teachers learned the names of the students whose hands were always up!

When you're hard pressed, it may seem easier just to get on with the job by yourself. Why should you take on the extra work of chasing them when they don't return calls or follow through the things they agreed to do? Your frustration is understandable but remember that working as a team almost always gets better results because it allows you to draw on a much wider range of skills and experience.

It can also act as a check if you get too close to the situation – as I have often done – and are not always able to see clearly the way things actually are or could be. If they don't return your calls don't give up but keep trying – as one social worker told me, 'It's the creaky gate that gets oiled.'

Tips on Being a Good Team Player

- Keep a note of all the useful names and telephone numbers in your notebook and mobile phone.
- If you have a computer, it's a good idea to keep a 'master document' with the names, roles and contact details for each of the professionals. Giving them a copy of this document – by email or on paper – can save the professionals a lot of time and be really helpful.
- Always make sure that you have a printed list of all the medications with you whenever you attend any medical or medical-related appointment about your loved one. Keeping a master document of medications on your computer makes this easy.
- If you are concerned about anything, don't leave it until Friday to call.
- Try and find out who in the 'care team' talks to whom and what arrangements there are for information to be shared.
- If you don't understand something, ask them to explain again.
- Don't allow people to rush you; you're entitled to ask for time to think things through or find out more.
- Take up any offers of help.

- Remember most professionals go into the work because they *do* care. Just like you, they get frustrated when form-filling, legislation and overload get in the way of them doing what they originally signed up for – making people's lives fractionally easier.

What to do if you hit a brick wall

'Social workers are key to accessing most things and if you don't get on with who you have been allocated, ask for a different one. It is not a problem to the social workers and they may actually be relieved if they are struggling to get on with you! It is so important that you get help and this relies on being able to express your needs, which you will only feel comfortable doing with someone you feel you can trust, or who is on your wavelength.'

Jill

You may be lucky enough to meet only warm and wonderful professionals who support you and the person you care for with skills, commitment and understanding.

But since we live in the real world it's likely that occasionally you'll reach a dead end or run smack into a brick wall.

If on your journey through the maze you encounter confusion, delays, lack of understanding or worse, don't be afraid to bring in other professionals to help you find a way through. Carers centres, your 'case worker', the Citizen's Advice Bureau, Age UK or even your own doctor may be able to succeed where you've been making no headway. There are more suggestions for organisations to turn to in the resources section at the back of this book.

If the worst comes to the worst, every organisation you rub shoulders with while you are caring will have its own complaints and appeals process, which those same people can help you to navigate.

The other tool that may help you is learning to be more assertive; how to stand your ground and push – in the nicest possible way – for what you want. Assertiveness is not about bad manners or being aggressive; it's about valuing yourself and your opinions as much as you value those of others, and it's about expressing your thoughts, feelings and beliefs in a straightforward, honest and appropriate way.

A Crash Course in Being Assertive

- Use 'I' messages. 'I find it hard to plan my day because I never know what time you're coming' is more effective than 'You're always late' which will put them on the defensive.
- Use facts rather than judgements. 'I have been waiting for you to get back to me as we agreed at our last meeting' rather than 'You seem to be forgetting or ignoring us.'
- Own your feelings – it's much more powerful. 'I'm angry that they made this decision without me' rather than 'They've made me angry.'
- Use direct words – 'no' rather than 'I don't think so', 'yes' rather than 'if you possibly can'.
- Make sure your expression matches your message and maintain eye contact. Sometimes when we're feeling awkward, we smile or look away even though what we're saying is serious.
- Keep your voice firm but pleasant.

- Write down the key points you want to make and practise them in advance so you can stay focused.
- Keep your posture open and relaxed which will help you speak clearly and strongly.
- Listen carefully to any response and let them know you've heard what they said.
- Don't be scared to keep repeating your point if they don't seem to be hearing you.

Keeping records

I've said this before, but it bears repeating here in light of my point that you can't always count on the other members of the care team to talk to you or each other. Every time you have a conversation, find something out, make an appointment or get a call from someone, jot it down. You should also make a note of what's been agreed, new information, names, dates and telephone numbers, as well as keeping records of tests, results, anything new or unusual affecting your loved one, and so on.

What this means is that at least one person is connecting up all the dots. It also means if someone fails to spot something, forgets to do something they've agreed, or needs information to help make an important decision, you have the evidence they need.

While I hesitate to ask you to do their job on top of the two or three jobs you are already doing as a carer, my justification is that this is about saving *you* time, frustration and heartache.

Finally, just in case you should ever need to go into battle with the professionals, you have a precise record of what was agreed, when and by whom.

CHAPTER 5

Money Matters

Some of us find it hard to get our heads around the subject of money so, to simplify things, I'm making this chapter *mainly* about money matters relating to the person you are caring for, and the benefits system for you both. In the next chapter, we'll look in more detail at *your* finances. I'll also be signposting you to some of the sources of financial support.

Paying for services

We've already looked, in the chapter on assessments, at the fact that if you are caring for an adult they may have to make some contribution towards the cost of any social care they receive.

It's an area where more change is likely as pressures on health and social care budgets become even greater. And there are differences even within the four nations of the UK. So for this reason I am going to focus only on the headlines of paying for care. For the most up-to-date information on payment thresholds – when people are and are no longer required to contribute to their care – see https://carers.org or www.carersuk.org.

The Government determines the minimum income it thinks any of us needs to live on. Even if your loved one is only receiving that minimum, it's likely they'll still be asked to contribute a nominal sum; for instance, towards visits to a day centre or paid carers coming in.

If your loved one has savings or other assets above a not-particularly-generous threshold, they are likely to be liable for all or most of their social care costs. They will do this until their savings drop below that threshold, at which point their contributions start to decrease.

If their savings fall below an even lower threshold, which represents about the combined cost of paying for a funeral and replacing the central heating system, your loved one is allowed to hang on to them.

Knowing which benefits are available

Knowing how tough it is for carers, you might expect the authorities to at least alert you to the fact that you might be able to get some financial help. Sadly, most carers tell a different story, like Mary whose daughter had severe learning difficulties and was given a place at a special school. Mary recalls, 'Because we lived a long way from the school, I didn't meet the other parents until one of the teachers arranged a coffee morning and that was when one of the other mums mentioned carer's allowance. I said, "Excuse me, what's that?" The others said, "Aren't you getting it?" So of course I applied and the next time I saw my GP I told him and he looked a bit awkward and said, "Oh, I always assumed you were ... being a professional I thought you'd know about it."'

The section below on what you're entitled to outlines some of the main benefits you may be able to apply for – either for your loved one, for you, or in some cases for both of you. It's not comprehensive – the rules for each benefit run into pages just by themselves. And rules about eligibility and amounts change so often, it's always best to check the current position.

A further complication is that there are different rules depending on where you live: what you can apply for and what you'll get varies according to whether you are in England, Northern Ireland, Scotland or Wales.

Use the list as a guide only – and make time to use one of the online benefits calculators at www.entitledto.co.uk or www.turn2us.org.uk. These are an excellent source for signposting you to the benefits you and your loved one are most likely to qualify for.

As always, the nearest carers centre or CAB will also be right up to speed on benefits and qualifying for them. If you are feeling even the slightest bit overwhelmed then start this process by talking to them.

Details of these services and others assisting with money matters are given in the resources section at the back of this book. Not only will they be able to tell you what you may qualify for but they can help you fill out cumbersome forms and collect together the evidence you'll need to make each claim.

The other important aspect of claiming financial help that such agencies can help you with is how the mish-mash of allowances and benefits affect each other. You don't want to go through all the pain of applying only to find out that what the Government gives with one hand it will remove with the other – something which is especially true for those carers who decide they want to continue to work.

On the other hand, qualifying for certain benefits can sometimes trigger other benefits and allowances automatically.

What could you and your loved one be entitled to?

There are benefits just for carers, some for people with a disability, and some to help you if you have a low income. Remember, you can still claim some benefits if you work, have savings or own your own home.

- You may be able to claim **Carer's Allowance** if you are caring for someone for 35 hours a week or more. Don't get excited – it's always been a paltry sum, but you can claim it alongside other benefits. And qualifying for it may increase the amounts you receive in other benefits.

- The person you care for may be able to get help with the extra costs of being disabled or having a long-term health condition. The benefits to check first are:

  ○ **Attendance Allowance** – if they are over 65, attendance allowance is intended to help towards the extra costs which are due to your loved one's condition. It is *not* means tested; there are two flat rates depending on how seriously ill or disabled they are.

  ○ **Personal Independence Payment** – if the person you care for is aged 16–64 then they may qualify for PIP as a contribution towards their living costs. It involves an assessment by a health professional who will determine how much they get depending on how their condition affects them.

- Both of you could qualify for **tax credits**, **income support** or **pension credits** if your total income falls below a set minimum. The rules on these depend where in the UK you live, your age and whether you are still working.

- Again, depending on income, you, your loved one, or both of you if you are living together, may qualify for **housing benefit** and to have your **council tax** paid in full or partially.

- If you are on low incomes, you and your loved one may qualify for help with **health costs,** such as dental treatment and prescriptions. Certain medical conditions will also qualify your loved one for free prescriptions if they are under 60. Beyond that age, they are free anyway. The NHS has a **Healthcare Travel Costs Scheme** (HTCS) reimbursing reasonable travel expenses to and from hospital appointments for both the patient and, in some circumstances, the carer.

- You may be able to apply for extra money from **grants** or **ben-evolent funds**, or get money off your **TV licence** or **car tax.** There's a lot more information on this, and likely sources for one-off support, on both https://carers.org and www.carersuk.org.
- There are **bereavement benefits** available to help those on low incomes when someone dies.

Other sources of support

Some social services departments or health authorities may give financial help towards the cost of buying special equipment or making significant changes to the house where you do your caring – for instance, widening doors or installing a wet room – so be sure to ask.

Councils may also make minor works grants at their own discretion, or this may be arranged through the occupational therapy service so it pays to talk to them before you lay out any cash.

The Family Fund distributes money in the form of one-off grants to support low-income families caring for anyone under the age of 16 at home who has a severe disability or is seriously ill. This is to assist with the costs of items such as play equipment, washing machines and dryers and holidays.

The charity sector is another source to consider if you are struggling to afford things that will have a positive effect on the quality of life and care you can provide. A number of charities may help you get away on holiday, with the person you're caring for, or for them alone so you can get some respite.

A few of the charities set up to support people with particular conditions have special funds to assist people in hardship, as do some of the unions and professional associations the person you're caring for might once have belonged to.

Other sources to consider are the ex-Forces organisations such as SSAFA, fundraising groups such as the Masons, and local philanthropic trusts. These are the hardest to locate since some of them try *not* to promote themselves in case they're besieged with more applications than they can cope with.

But your local library is a good place to enquire and will almost certainly keep a copy of the *Directory of Grant Making Trusts* in the reference section.

To apply or not to apply

As a carer and a coper, I'm willing to bet that the very idea of asking for money is a tough one for you. You certainly won't be the first to think that if our society valued carers it would make sure they were financially OK without any carer ever having to ask for help.

And then there are those of you who've already tried asking for help and encountered enough suspicion and red tape to leave a seriously bad taste in your mouth. At which point your thinking goes something like: 'Well, if you're going to make it so damn hard then forget it. I'll just get on and do the job without you, same as I have been doing for the last umpteen years.' Your anger and frustration are understandable but, before you tear the forms into tiny pieces, you should know that carers currently save the economy around £132 billion a year – around £20,000 a head.

I have yet to meet a carer who wouldn't go the extra mile for someone in the same boat as themselves. Every time one of us takes on the system and wins a bit of cash or recognition it shifts officialdom's understanding of a carer's life a few inches forward. Not much, I'll agree, but somewhere down the line, we'll have all travelled far enough for change to come. And you'll have done your bit to make that happen.

Looking after someone else's money

If you are caring for an adult who is, or becomes, physically unable to leave the house, or mentally unable to manage their own affairs, you may have to get involved in looking after their finances for them.

Not surprisingly, something which our society sets so much store by can prove to be a minefield for the best-intentioned carer. To the one you care for, handing over control of their finances to someone else may underline their dependency more than anything else. And if they have lived through hard times, and struggled to manage their own money carefully, seeing it in someone else's hands can make them feel especially vulnerable.

While this is going on, you may have other people's issues to take account of, too, like Peter who felt other family members were suspicious of him taking charge of a great aunt's money for her. Peter recalls, 'It was me going in there every day to clean up and water the garden and take her into town so we could pay her bills. She was confused and I'd often pay for things then she'd forget to pay me back. That was why it hurt so much when word reached me our aunt was telling other people she didn't know where her money was going. No one said anything but I felt fingers were being pointed. It was ironic, given how much it was costing me to be a carer!'

Before such situations develop, it's a good idea, if you possibly can, to get together everyone involved for a family conference to discuss managing your relative's money. The last thing you need is to have to worry about what others might be saying. Who knows, it might even be an opportunity to enlist help from them. They could share the load by taking charge of some of the book-keeping or bill-paying.

Below, we'll look at a few of the areas where you may get involved in helping someone else with their money.

Bank and savings accounts

The simplest way to make withdrawing and depositing money easy for you both is to open a joint account, or alter their existing bank or building society account so you are both named on it. This has the added advantage that should your loved one be too unwell to get at their money, or should they die, you, as a shareholder in the account, would still have access to the money for direct expenses. Meanwhile, you both get to see the balance and statements so you can feel reassured that everything is out in the open.

If you don't want to go that far, the person you care for can ask the bank or building society to make you an authorised user of their account by giving you what's known as a 'third-party mandate'.

Online banking is another option that is quick, convenient, and lets you see how their finances stand without having to contact anyone or request a statement. However, for some people, dealing with their finances via the hubbub of the Internet is a leap of faith too far.

Lasting Power of Attorney

I know you are already suffering death by form-filling but there's no getting away from the importance of this one. While the person you care for still has what is defined as 'capacity' – the ability to understand decisions they need to make, why they need to make them and the likely consequences of those decisions – do encourage them to set up a Lasting Power of Attorney (LPA) with your help.

An LPA allows someone to act and make decisions on their behalf if they are no longer able to do so. There are two types – for property and financial affairs, and for health and welfare – but in this chapter it's looking after the money and financial affairs of the person you care for that we're concerned about.

The most important piece of advice I have for you under the category of money is to encourage your loved one to apply for an LPA at the earliest opportunity, even if they are still managing well. I have heard stories from people who didn't do this and ended up having to take out personal loans to cover the cost of care while they sorted out getting access to the money of someone who had lost capacity or the ability to manage their own finances. (And, by the way, one tactic for encouraging your loved one to set up an LPA is to do it for yourself at the same time. It's never too soon to do this as insurance against a future none of us can predict.)

You can download or complete the forms online from the Office of the Public Guardian, or by visiting the relevant section of the UK Government website; see the resources section at the back of this book.

It's worth just noting that up to 2007, when the LPA came in, some people set up an Enduring Power of Attorney (EPA). EPAs made and signed before 1 October 2007 should still be valid but cover decisions about only property and financial affairs.

A number of organisations such as CAB and Age UK publish resources on dealing with someone else's money, so do check those out.

If this advice comes too late and the person you care for 'lacks mental capacity', you can still apply to the Office of the Public Guardian to become their 'deputy' in order to handle their affairs. This would allow you to deal with, for example, their bank and care providers.

However, if their income comprises only a state pension and/or welfare benefits, and there is no LPA, rather than applying to become a deputy you can apply directly to the Department of Work and Pensions to become an appointee – which will allow you to receive and pay out income on their behalf. This same route can apply to benefits that come from their local council, such as housing or council tax benefit.

Making a Will

Making a Will is another area where you may feel wary to tread, but if the person you're caring for is elderly or suffering from a terminal illness it's wise to ensure their wishes are formally recorded so they have the status of law when they die. This is particularly important if you're sharing their home or own property or other assets, such as a car, jointly. You need to know where you'll stand if they die.

Because of your close relationship with the person you're caring for, it's probably a good idea to pay for the Will to be drawn up independently by a solicitor. In the UK, look out for Free Will Weeks, when in return for a nominal donation to a charity in the Will, a solicitor will draw up a simple Will free of charge.

Think carefully with your loved one about who should be named as executors of the Will – the people whose job it is to see the wishes in the Will are 'executed' or carried out. Some people choose to make the solicitor who helped draw up the Will one of the executors. If there isn't much in the way of assets, you may find it all goes in solicitors' fees rather than to the people or causes that your loved one intended.

On the other hand, having a 'neutral' person as an executor should be proof against a situation where the Will was drawn up some time before and, because life rarely stands still, the executors chosen at the time are, for one reason or another, no longer able to act themselves.

As with all money affairs, it's a good idea to get independent advice from a reputable financial adviser.

Practicalities

- Have the money conversations as soon as you can – the longer you leave it the more awkward you are going to feel.
- Sit down with your loved one and write a list of the most

important information you are going to need: account numbers for banks, savings accounts, utilities and any other services where money changes hands, passwords, where they keep statements, and their Will.

● Establish who is going to have access to what and, as much as you can, keep this information in the open between you, them and any other close family members who need to be informed.

Difficult conversations

All of this is very well, but doesn't take account of those of you whose loved ones would rather have all their teeth extracted than talk about money. Or who simply don't see the need to act while they are still feeling well.

This is when it might be helpful to bring in one of the professionals, to explain what needs to happen and why – in order that you can help them. We're all familiar with the effect an official uniform or title can have on our willingness to go along with something so it's worth a try.

Another route that has worked for some carers is doing this financial housekeeping in tandem with their loved one; bringing in a solicitor to talk through and produce a Power of Attorney, Wills and a financial plan for both them *and* you.

Controlling spending

'Mum had always been so tight with money, refusing to have coffee out when she could make it for a few pence at home. After her stroke, she changed out of all recognition. There was this pile of mail-order catalogues alongside her chair and packages of stuff she'd no use for arriving every day. I was desperate, worrying she'd run out of money.'

Rose

It's one thing to spend the children's inheritance, and quite another when your loved one starts acting completely out of character, putting their own financial well-being at risk as Rose's mother did.

Nor is it uncommon. Contributors to one carers' forum reported finding their loved ones had been stockpiling everything from tinned vegetables to outdoor shoes. One carer told me her relative's home resembled the 'before' on one of the TV shows about hoarders. In amongst our mum's things, we counted more than two hundred bars of soap.

So how do you deal with a dramatic change in your loved one's ability to manage their money?

- As much as you can, keep temptation out of reach. Avoid shops when you make excursions.
- Bring in a cash-only regime if you can, with an agreed amount in their purse or wallet each week – once it's gone, it's gone.
- Intercept at least some of the catalogues and send them back with 'gone away' written across your loved one's address.
- Make sure they are ex-directory and registered with both the telephone preference service www.tpsonline.org.uk (which is supposed to stop at least some of the cold calls) and the mail preference service www.mpsonline.org.uk (which should stop at least some of the junk mail).

CHAPTER 6

More on Money – Help for You As a Carer

'When my daughter, Sophie, fell ill and needed full-time care, the last thing on my mind was my career or a salary. But now, six years later, I cannot ignore how drastically her disability has affected my life and income. Although I am not poor, luxuries that I could afford easily before have become a distant memory . . . Even with a comprehensive care package in place, it is impossible to overestimate the financial implications of having a member of the family who needs full-time home care.'

Judith Cameron, 'Who Cares?'
blogpost for the *Guardian*, 6 June 2005

The high cost of caring

Judith is not alone. On top of everything else carers have to worry about, figures from Carers UK in 2016 reveal 44 per cent of carers struggling to make ends meet, while Carers Trust report 60 per cent of carers have used all their savings to cover the costs of caring.

When you factor in that £132 billion contribution carers are making – around one fifth of UK Government spending – it's hard to escape the conclusion that carers are effectively subsidising the state.

As a carer, you face the double whammy of your income dropping if you give up your job or go part-time in order to care, while at the same time your expenses are rocketing. For example, it's estimated that the everyday cost of raising a disabled child is three times that of bringing up a non-disabled youngster because of the extra equipment and services required.

Additional childcare for you, transportation, wear and tear; these are the hidden costs of caring. And they are only the tip of a frightening iceberg. If you're at home all day, and especially if the person you care for is frail or unwell, you may need to keep your heating on during the eight months of the year when it's not warm.

If you're trying to juggle caring with running your own home, with paid work, with family responsibilities, and it's 9 p.m. before you're free to sit down and eat, then expensive ready meals may be your only option.

Shortage of time can force you to make other choices which come at a higher cost: doing your shopping online which means paying for it to be delivered, or picked up from the closest convenience store rather than the cheap supermarket five miles and two bus rides down the road; bringing in a cleaner because you can't even manage a lick and a promise; or, when you get two hours' rare respite, calling a taxi to take you into town because if you wait for a bus then half your time is gone.

Then add to your budget the additional costs of any aids and equipment you may need to buy your loved one for which – with the best will in the world – you won't always be reimbursed: clothes that are easy to get on and off; a higher bed or chair; safety guards; extra incontinence pads. And what about the washing bill if the person you care for needs clean sheets every day? The list is endless.

If the person you are caring for is receiving attendance allowance then do remember this isn't intended to be 'pocket money' for them but to reimburse these additional expenses that go with the territory – *including yours* – for all those things I've just listed.

Your pension

If you're still of working age, you'll want to think about protecting your pension while you are caring. As with the other benefits we've discussed, the rules on this do change from time to time. The important thing to know is that your pension depends on your National Insurance contributions so, if you give up work to care for someone, then it's important to check whether your NI contributions will be automatically paid for you. If you receive certain benefits such as carer's allowance, they will be. But do talk to your nearest carers centre, consult one of the carers organisation websites, or talk directly to the Government's own benefits hotline to check your personal position.

Get financially savvy

Accessing some of the benefits I covered in the previous chapter may help a fraction. But let's not pretend the benefits system aims to do more than keep the wolf from the door. Moreover, if you are working part-time, it's quite possible to find yourself earning just enough to put you fractionally on the wrong side of the state's safety net.

When it comes to money, some of us prefer to bury our heads in the sand and hope things will work out somehow. But it does pay to bite the bullet and learn enough to ensure you will be OK financially.

There are plenty of books and blogs you can find to guide you through money literacy. Two I like are:

- A free Open University course on 'Managing my Money': http://www.open.edu/openlearn/money-management/managing-my-money/content-section-overview
- A free service from Barclays bank which has learning modules for a range of circumstances and financial needs: https://financial.wings.uk.barclays/

Tips from carers

Another strategy is to make what you do have stretch as far as possible, and ensure managing your finances is as convenient and efficient as it can be. I'm not going to suggest you cut out the occasional cup of coffee with a friend, or other treats. You need them and you deserve them. But these money-saving tips have come from other carers:

- Cancel all but one credit card. It's useful to have one for ordering online or on the phone and for when you're not carrying much cash. Having one means only one bill and you can keep track better of how much you're racking up on it.
- Or make it a strict rule that you have one credit card for expenditure related only to your loved one and a separate one that is *never* used for your loved one so you can keep a firm grip on both.
- Put absolutely everything you can on to direct debit. It feels like you're giving up control but in return you know that the same amount is going out of your account every month of the year. There'll be no horrible surprises and you can budget properly knowing what you've got left for the rest of the month.
- Few companies reward loyalty. You won't have time to do all the research on getting cheaper deals for everything from fuel and insurance to phone and broadband. But if you sign up for a reputable comparison site like www.moneysavingexpert.com they'll do the donkey work for you. They may also help identify

those companies that offer discounts for older or disabled customers.

- If you have a car, could you manage with a smaller engine that will use less fuel, or, when friends ask what they can do to help, suggest they give you lifts in their car?
- Investigate small savings that add up to more significant sums. As the carer of someone with mobility problems, you may be exempt from car tax which frees up another £2 a week.
- You can also try the 'separate purses' or jam jar approach, where you have different physical places to keep money for separate purposes. When it's gone, it's gone.
- If you've had to give up work, do you have any office or practical skills you could use to earn a little extra from home?
- If you think your need for money may be short- to medium-term and you own your own home, you could consider re-mortaging to free up some cash and reduce your monthly payments.
- Keep a record of all your spending for at least a week. Be religious about it and write down absolutely everything. It will help you spot any areas where you could make savings and any unhelpful patterns such as spending to make yourself feel better.

CHAPTER 7

Working through It – Carers and the World of Work

'Something had to give and that something turned out to be work. One day I thought, "That's it ... I'm off." I said to myself, "I'll have a year off," but Mum got used to me being there and, after a year, I realised I couldn't leave her.'

Janet

'Endless energy, excellent communication and negotiating skills, the ability to stay calm under pressure, to make good decisions, juggle and prioritise competing demands, work independently and remain motivated ...' This sounds like the perfect person spec that employers would snap up. Actually, these are just a few of the qualities carers are called on to exhibit every day of their lives.

For many of us being a carer feels like a full-time job. Yet the 2011 census found around three million people – one in nine of the UK workforce – combine caring with paid employment.

Herding cats doesn't come close to the challenge of managing two sets of competing – and usually very different – demands. And that's before you've also tried to fit in the rest of your life: family, friends, hobbies, health, 'you' time . . .

Some decide the only way to cope is to stop trying and give up the 'day job'. According to Carers Trust, one in five carers give up employment to care. Others slog on, helped or hindered by their employers.

Like so much to do with being a carer, there are rarely easy choices. If you do give up paid employment, will you be able to cope on the miserly carer's allowance and other benefits? How easy will it be to get back into work should circumstances change? How much of your personal fulfilment comes from the work you do?

But if you stay, will your career suffer because you haven't the energy to give the job your all? Will you be thought less committed if you're always having to dash off to deal with emergencies?

Before you make any decisions, you need time to find out precisely what your choices are. What are your legal rights? How flexible is your employer willing to be? How much help can you get?

A little help from the law

Growing awareness of people's changing needs is slowly percolating through to politicians and legislators with the result that even unsympathetic employers may now find themselves bound by law to respond to your request for flexibility. Below are a few of the headlines. However, do use the resources section at the end of this book to check out the latest position.

- If you've been with your current employer for six months or more then you have the right to request flexible working (skip forward to 'employers who care' to see some of the ways in which carers have made this work for them).

- Employees now have the right to take a 'reasonable' amount of time off work to deal with an emergency involving a dependent. However, it is up to your employer whether that time is paid or unpaid.
- If you've been with your employer for twelve months and you are responsible for a child aged under 18, you are entitled to 18 weeks leave per child, which must be taken by the child's 18th birthday. Again, this may well be unpaid.
- You are protected by a range of legislation from discrimination on the grounds of your role as a carer.
- And the Carers Equal Opportunities Act 2004 and Equality Act 2010 say local authorities must take carers' wishes about work, education and training into account when they carry out their carer's assessment. So if you decide you want to go on working the care plan needs to set out how your loved one will be looked after while you're at work.

Employers who care

Some carers choose not to say anything at all to their employer or colleagues, for fear of being thought unreliable, less committed, or too big a risk when it comes to promotion. The choice is up to you. But the world of work is changing and, for every employer still stuck in the Dark Ages, there are far more employers that now recognise the importance of a healthy work-life balance, who don't expect staff to leave their personal lives with their coats at the front door, and who understand that recruiting and retaining good staff means meeting them halfway when it comes to flexibility.

The fact that 60 per cent of us will be carers at some point in our working lives has helped drive the shift towards more family-friendly policies. That's an awful lot of experience and skill to lose if the world of work doesn't find ways to accommodate today's complicated lives.

Being a flexible employer might mean anything from allowing you to use the phone for personal calls, to granting unpaid leave, renegotiating hours, or allowing you to do more work from home.

Ros's employer twice adjusted her hours so she could continue to work and care. She explains, 'I was working full-time so we agreed I'd start at 7 a.m. so I could take a three-hour lunchbreak to see Mum and sort out her meal and the house. Because I was going to her after work, too, the days were just too long. I was only getting a few hours' sleep each night so they agreed to reduce my hours to give me enough time to do the lunchtime visit without the early start. It's on a six-month renewable basis; I didn't want to make permanent changes in case I need to go back full-time.'

A number of well-known business names are leading the way and have formed an action group, Employers for Carers, to offer advice and support to other companies and to carers. Among the solutions they suggest are:

- **'compress'** your day – start and finish early, or start and finish late, so you have time at one end of the day to meet your caring responsibilities.
- **'stretch'** your day by taking a two- or three-hour lunch breaks to be a carer before returning to work.
- **'extend'** your working week – spread your hours over six days, giving you shorter hours each working day.
- go part-time, work only term-time, or organise a job share.
- negotiate an allowance of unpaid leave so you don't have to use your entire holiday entitlement on being a carer.
- join the growing army of remote or home workers whose employers have provided the equipment for them to do more work from home.

Bear in mind, too, that apart from your legal rights, your employer may have its own carer-friendly policies; these may even form part of their employment contract with you. If you're not sure, then consult the personnel or human resources team, a trade union or professional association, or your line manager, to see how your employer provides for carers. And if they don't currently, see if they are willing to sit down and discuss your terms and conditions to enable you to continue to work while you are a carer. You can point them to www.employersforcarers.org for advice and support.

Deciding whether to stay or go

At a time when so much is out of your hands, when events seem simply to be happening *to* you, giving yourself the breathing space to make an informed choice is a way of helping you feel just a little more in control. Use the checklist below to structure your thinking and to help you talk your options through with your employer, and with those you trust and who know you well.

- What are your options at work? How flexible is your employer? Would a few simple changes to your hours or conditions make a dramatic difference?
- If there really aren't enough hours in the day, would working part-time (or further reducing your hours if you're already part-time) work for you and your employer? Is job-sharing a possibility?
- Do you have any idea how long your role as a carer will last? If the person you're caring for is terminally ill, could you negotiate the kind of career break offered to new parents?
- If you stay, what will be the effects of doing two jobs on your health and well-being? Are you the kind of person who will feel more stressed because you're worrying you're not doing either job properly?

- Have you done the sums to see whether you can manage on less money?
- How would giving up work or cutting your hours affect your pension? Does your employer's scheme allow payment 'holidays', or can you continue to make payments privately?
- Depending on the kind of work you're in, will your skills quickly get out of date?
- Finally, how important is your paid work to you? Are you someone who needs to be involved and feeling useful? To what extent is your self-esteem tied to being good at your job?

Staying employable

But what if you try to negotiate a flexible package and get nowhere? Or your caring role is so onerous you feel you have no choice but to pack up the paid portion of your working week?

Before you depart, do explore whether you can get a little extra cash behind you by negotiating your departure on different terms; for instance, by taking voluntary redundancy or even early retirement.

If you're likely to want to return to paid work some time – whether to your old employer or pastures new – see if you can set up a few systems to stay in touch. Is there a staff or professional newsletter whose mailing list you could go on? Could your former colleagues let you know about any events you could attend? Or allow you to access the staff Intranet or even occasional training days?

There may also be local networks in your field of work. Talk to your local library, chamber of commerce, or branch of your union or professional association.

And don't forget the infinite resources of the Internet.

- Many colleges and universities now offer distance learning courses for professional updating or retraining. The Open

University and Open College led the way in these and changes in adult education funding mean, if you're not working, you've got the same entitlement to a student loan as school leavers, with repayments delayed until you are earning over a set sum.

- Or check out some of the places offering free online courses listed in the resources section at the back of this book.
- If you're returning to work there are local agencies who can help with everything from professional refresher courses to job hunting and preparing a CV. Talk to your carers centre, CAB, job centre or library for signposting to these.

One issue that many carers mentioned to me is the effect giving up paid work has had on their self-esteem. At a time when your identity is often taking a hammering from a role which requires you to park many of your own needs, hanging on to your sense of who you are and what you're worth can be really tough. Staying in touch with the 'you' who operates successfully in the outside world of work may help keep your self-esteem intact.

Being a carer is a job, too

If you have given up your job – even temporarily – try to remind yourself often of the skills and experience your new role demands. And don't forget that in choosing to be a carer, you are exhibiting qualities such as loyalty and commitment – qualities that are on every employer's 'shopping list'. The job ad below may get you thinking about how many skills and qualities you do have, and you could consider using some of these words in a future job application.

Are You up to the Challenge of Being a Carer?

We're looking for an exceptional person for this vital role. As a carer, your efforts will guarantee a high quality of life for those in most need.

- You'll need boundless energy, huge stamina, and an ability to work under pressure.
- Your role will bring you into contact with a wide range of official and voluntary agencies so you'll need excellent communication, negotiation and listening skills.
- You should be able to juggle half-a-dozen tasks at any time, all of them important, without getting flustered.
- It's essential that you're able to prioritise your workload, have the ability to make decisions quickly, and can work independently, without supervision or regular support.
- You'll have bucketloads of patience and understanding, remain motivated even when you feel you're not getting any help or recognition, and be flexible about time off (we're not able to offer much).
- Finally, a sense of humour is essential.

CHAPTER 8

Home Sweet Home

'It doesn't matter how big your house is, how remote the annex is or how thick the walls are, you'll still be able to hear their TV. It will be on all of the time and Flog It, Countdown and Gardeners' World will become the background soundtrack to your every waking moment.'

Anonymous contributor to Age Space:
www.agespace.org/10-things-no-one-tells-you

'Home sweet home' . . . 'home is where the heart is' . . . 'there's no place like home' . . . for many of us, home is supposed to be the place we go to escape from the pressures of the world, to take a deep breath, to be ourselves. Whether you move in with them or they come and live with you, caring for another adult under the same roof will change the way you think about home. From being a sanctuary, it is transformed into a workplace, a pressure cooker, even a prison, no matter how much you love the person you're caring for.

Anything you can do to make home work better for you both, to keep it safe, to find space in it for a bit of sanctuary, will be worth the effort. Let's look at how.

The 'where' of care

*'I always knew I needed to be able to escape behind my own
front door. We moved Mum into the cottage next door and
I was there first thing, last thing and often during the day.
But those twenty steps it took me to go from one front door to
another were my lifeline.'*

Kate

Of the millions of carers living under the same roof as the person
they care for, almost nine in every ten will be doing so in their own
home. That figure, of course, includes parents caring for a child –
often more than one – with special needs. Of the remainder, the
majority are single adults, caring for a parent in the family home.

Geography, or your relationship to the person you care for, may have
already made the 'where to care' decision for you – we'll say more
about caring at a distance in a moment. But there are situations
where you have a choice. And if so, it's important to think through
how each possibility will impact on your life as well as your ability
to care.

Here are some of the things to think about, whether you're new to
caring, or reviewing a situation that doesn't seem to be working.

- What's your relationship like with the person you're caring
  for? Illness or dependency can change the dynamics of our
  relationships, but not always for the better, particularly if you've
  struggled spending too much time together in the past.
- How much care do they need? If you're always being summoned
  by alarm calls at night would it be less wearing on you if you only
  need put on a dressing gown rather than drive across town?
- What impact is caring having on your finances? Once you've
  looked into what you and they are entitled to, could you save
  money by sharing one home rather than running two?

- Are there other people to consider? Will your own partner and children be able to cope if the person you are caring for comes to live with you? Or if you go to live with them, will that be an excuse for other siblings, partners and family to step back?
- How important to your loved one's well-being are familiar surroundings, the chance to keep a much-loved pet for instance? The ability to stay in touch with local neighbours and friends?
- Same question to you: if you move in with them, are you cutting yourself off from your support networks? And will there be somewhere to escape to in their home – a room of your own? If they have to go into a nursing home or if they die, will you still have a home?
- What about the practicalities? Do you have enough space? Can the home be adapted for care?
- If you're caring for a partner, has it become important to move out of a shared bedroom and create a space of your own?
- Are you really facing an either/or decision? Are there other options, like Kate's above, moving close to each other without being under the same roof? Or is the best decision to secure a place for them in the right residential setting – supported living through to care and nursing homes? See Chapter 16 for more on making decisions regarding residential care.

It's unlikely there'll be a 'perfect' solution. But you stand the best chance of success if you remember that your own needs must be part of your decision-making if this is to work for you both.

The special challenges of caring at a distance

'Mum and I spoke on the phone every Sunday but she seemed so well I never thought of organising an alarm button or phoning more often. Only when I couldn't get hold of her one Sunday, I panicked. We called relatives in the same town who called the

police to break in. She'd had a massive stroke two days before.
It still gives me nightmares to think of her lying on the floor,
getting colder and more scared, within sight of the phone but no
more capable of reaching it than of flying to the moon. What if
she'd had the stroke on a Monday rather than Friday?'

Tom

One of the challenges of distance is knowing what is *really* going on.
It wasn't until we were moving Mum from the huge house where
she lived alone to stay with us temporarily that we really noticed she
might not have been coping. Every room was clogged with stuff she'd
bought through mail order and never opened.

Other carers say it was only when a crisis occurred that they came
across mountains of unpaid bills, and different mountains of dust
and dirt. Of course, this may not happen to you; you may even, like
me, want to believe your loved one is coping well because you know
how important their independence is to them – and, if I'm honest,
to your ability to live your life. But if you suspect your loved one(s)
of being expert at putting on a front, then it may be an idea to call in
occasionally at times when you're not expected.

Not knowing what's going on is only one of the challenges, however.
There's also the time and money you'll be spending on travel, the fact
that you're possibly doubling your workload and expenses, looking
after two homes, cooking two lots of meals, paying two lots of bills.

Carol Lee's poignant account in *Out of Winter* of caring at a distance
for parents, living in Wales, that she had never felt close to, expresses
both the challenges and the rewards:

'It was an exhausting business. The 5 a.m. start for a blocked
drain in Wales, the shopping, cleaning, cooking, washing,
hospital appointments . . . and the beginnings of my mother's
short-term memory loss. I had my full life in London, too. The

*strain told in my weight loss, sleeplessness and the deep guilt
that I was never doing enough. The most important task of all
was the one I couldn't see at first – just being with them. "I feel so
safe and warm with you in the house," Mum said to me one night.'*

Working with the professionals also takes on an extra dimension
when you're dealing with health and social services in an area
different from your own, and needing extra time off for meetings
which are happening in another place.

On the other hand, you *do* get to go back to your own home sweet
home, and so do they. And because you are not immediately to hand,
social and health services will have to pick up a great deal more of
the slack once you've identified that your loved one can no longer
manage entirely alone.

The following checklist comes courtesy of the excellent
www.agespace.org website and will help you decide if the time
has come to intervene.

- Look around the house and garden to see if things are less well
  cared for than they used to be; is the house dirty, especially
  kitchen and bathroom? Is the laundry piling up?
- **Money** – are bills getting paid, or are there reminders in the post?
  If you are able to look at a bank statement, does it look like their
  spending patterns have changed?
- **Medication** – if they take medication, do they have a system for
  their pills and do they seem to be taking them regularly?
- **Personal hygiene** – are they wearing clean clothes and do they
  appear to be looking after themselves – hair, shaving, teeth? Can
  they still bath/shower?
- **Clothes** – are they over- or under-dressed for the weather?
- **Food** – check the fridge to make sure food is in date and to see if
  they appear to be eating regular meals. Are they still able to cook
  or heat food safely?

- **Mobility** – can they still get up and down stairs if they have them? Are they able to walk to shops or public transport, or to drive themselves safely?
- **Hobbies and socialising** – are they still doing the things they have enjoyed doing until now? Are they getting out to see friends or go to activities?

Need to know checklist

Wherever you're doing the caring, it's useful to know the following, but it takes on a special importance if you are not living with the person you care for.

- **Keys** – who has front door keys? Is there a spare set somewhere? Should there be a keysafe outside? Is there a burglar alarm and do you know the code? Where are the other keys – for the garage, garden shed, the desk where all the useful information may be stored?
- **Neighbours and friends** – do you have contact details for friends and neighbours who you can call on, particularly if you don't live close by?
- **Contact details** – have you got other important contacts, including doctor, adult social worker, and any care organisation that's involved?
- **Medical history** – a snapshot of important medical information such as the medicines they are on, allergies, chronic conditions and so on.
- **Passwords** – potentially a legal minefield because of data protection … but at the very least it is worth knowing the main login details and password to a computer, with details of any online accounts.
- **Finances** – bank account details, national insurance number, ID such as passport, driving licence, other important documents such as birth certificate, marriage certificate, Will, house and car insurance, service providers.

Making the environment work for you

By the time Mary's learning-disabled daughter had developed enough to walk, she'd outgrown the baby walkers aimed at helping tots stand on their own two feet. 'I decided to buy her a doll's pram instead and put a bag of cement in it so she could walk and it would support her,' Mary recalls.

Sometimes making daily life manageable is about this kind of ingenuity and experiment. Though there are literally hundreds of companies producing thousands of products to assist carers and those they care for, don't discount the possibility that the solution may be under your nose.

If you can, chat to others at support groups or via one of the many wonderfully reassuring online forums; you'll almost certainly find someone somewhere has already come up with a novel way of tackling the problem facing you.

As for professional help, the occupational therapist or district nurse should be able to offer lots of practical suggestions and may arrange to loan you equipment, or even help fund important adaptations to the home.

If you live in the town you may find a Disabled Living Centre or, if there isn't one locally, its parent body the Disabled Living Foundation, www.dlf.org.uk. These charities can advise on what the various appliances are actually called, as Caroline discovered. She said, 'There are some great websites out there for special equipment. Not knowing the names of things was a bit problem for me. For example, Dad and I both thought that he needed a white cane, but in fact this is the very long thing that requires specialist training to use. What he actually needed was a white walking stick. That took some finding out.'

The same sources can also advise on where to find second-hand equipment, put you in touch with suppliers and allow you to look at and test your options.

The list of equipment and adaptations you might consider is inexhaustible, with new ways to tackle common problems constantly under development – particularly in the use of technology to safeguard people in their own homes. The list below is intended only to give you a flavour of what's available and get you thinking about the sorts of things that might make life a fraction easier for you and your loved one in the home.

Common equipment and adaptations to consider

- **General** – long-handled catch openers for windows; pulleys for curtains; plugs with handles; raised electric sockets; entry and door ramps; community alarm system.
- **Hallway and stairs** – grab rails and/or bannisters along walls and doorways; stairlift; stairgate; night lights.
- **Living room** – remote controls for electrical equipment and lights; adjustable or high-seated chair; chair 'risers'; chair tray; mechanical grabber; speaker phone.
- **Bedroom** – electric adjustable bed; pressure mattress, support pillow, hoist or bed sticks to help them lift themselves in bed.
- **Bathroom and loo** – raised toilet seat; handrails; tap levers; bath or shower seat; walk-in bath or wet shower room; non-slip mats; long-handled brushes; liquid soap and shampoo dispensers; long-handled sponge or flannel stick.
- **Clothing** – long-handled shoe horn; gadget for putting on socks; dressing stick; simple fastenings such as Velcro.
- **Eating** – microwave; two-handled cup; plate guard; angled cutlery; bibs or aprons for everyone!
- **Telehealth** – personal alarms; passive infra-red (movement) detectors; fall detectors; property exit sensors and GPS; carbon monoxide, natural gas, smoke and flood detectors; panic buttons.

Crucially, these can not only be connected to a 24-hour alarm centre, but in most cases can also be monitored by carers.

While you're thinking about adaptations, bear in mind there's no reason the sitting room has to be where it's always been if converting it to a bedsit for your loved one would give them more independence and you a bit more space. Carers have turned laundry rooms into downstairs bathrooms, lounges into bedrooms, ground floors into first floors – whatever works for them. Even the smallest homes can be made a little more flexible with the introduction of a room divider.

And be aware that if you're buying aid items for your loved one to use then they are VAT exempt. The websites don't always make that clear because they're mainly selling to care providers who do have to pay VAT. Let them know when you buy that you are claiming the VAT exemption.

Getting organised

The following tips come from other carers who've found them useful for keeping on top of most things, most of the time:

- Create a bulletin board just for those things to do with caring: important telephone numbers, appointment cards, dietary details, whatever you and others need to be able to put your hands on instantly.
- Keep an extra set of those things that it would be disastrous to lose: keys, glasses, photocopies of important documents such as birth and marriage certificates, national insurance numbers, alarm codes, etc.
- Keep everything to do with the person you're caring for in a single accessible place such as an accordion file; for instance, details of medicines, treatments, their home, bills, finances, Will and so on. And if you're a computer user, have a master document with all these things in it that you can easily print out for a new professional.

- Display your phone number somewhere prominent in their home and/or in the ICE (in case of emergency) function on their mobile phone if they have one. You want to be reachable in an emergency. Consider investing in an SOS bracelet for yourself so if the emergency is yours, people quickly learn you are a carer and can activate the emergency plan for your loved one.

- Get an answerphone or set up voicemail on your mobile so you don't miss any crucial calls, but can also screen calls if you're shattered and don't feel like talking.

- Get a large wall calendar so neither of you miss any important appointments or visits – then get in the habit of consulting it every day.

- If their health is fragile, keep an overnight bag packed with essentials such as toothbrush, toiletries, nightwear – and something for you to read while you're doing the inevitable hanging around. And, most importantly, pack a copy of that printed list of current medication.

Staying safe

We're always being told more accidents happen in the home than anywhere else – and we're always being told it because it's true. Of course, you're already doing your best to keep you both safe but the busier our lives are, the more likely we are to overlook obvious things. As a carer with so much on your plate, you're more vulnerable.

Staying aware of safety means remembering some basic rules:

- Don't leave things lying on the floor, hallways or stairs where they will be trip hazards. Invest in a big straw basket and sling into it everything you need to put away but don't have time for right now.

- If you or your loved one has to get up at night, install a night light or put reflective tape on sharp corners and stair edges.

- A baby monitor is a simple way of staying aware of what else is going on in the house when you're tied up.
- Install smoke alarms if you haven't got them and change the batteries every New Year's Day, without fail.
- You may also want to invest in fire extinguishers and teach everyone in the house how to use them.
- The local fire brigade will do a free safety check, and that's also the opportunity for you to mention if your loved one is immobile or spends the majority of their time in a particular part of the house so they can have that information on record should the worst happen.
- Remove the lock on the bathroom door and hang an occupied sign on it instead. And consider rehanging the door so it opens outwards. This is now part of building regulations, so that if someone collapses against the door you can still get them out, but may not be the case in older properties.
- Get a community alarm pendant and system installed, so that in an emergency you or your loved one can notify someone immediately that you need help.
- And one vital rule for you: *slow down*. Whenever you find yourself rushing around the house, in the street, or behind the wheel of a car, actively tell yourself to 'slow down'. Seriously, rushing really doesn't get things done more quickly but it does raise your stress levels and put you at risk of accidents or mistakes that will only cause you more grief.

Creating a good environment for you both

And finally, we began this chapter with a reminder of what home means to us. More than ever for you as a carer it's important to preserve as much of that as you can.

If you are living with the person you care for, you need to think about what boundaries you can put in place to help you switch off sometimes. Having one room or a space in a room that is yours alone, for instance, filled with the things that make you feel good and at peace. It could be a bedroom, an attic conversion, even the garden shed, so long as going in and closing the door means you are temporarily off duty.

If your home's simply too small for that to be an option, think about how you can create mental boundaries. Your home is now, after all, your workplace. For most of us, the end of the working day involves at least a short journey home, which is a useful way of closing the door on the day. Could you take a turn round the block or the garden when the person you're caring for goes to bed? Or get into the habit of treating every bath you have or every meal you cook as time for you, surrounded with music you enjoy and good smells?

As your workplace, and an environment in which you are both spending a lot of time, you want the home to be not only practical but a really pleasant place to be. Think about the little touches that can help make it a place of peace and interest for you and put them on your Christmas or birthday list:

- wind chimes in a doorway or patio;
- house plants and, in the garden, perennials for year-round colour;
- a bird feeder outside the window or a low-maintenance pet such as goldfish;
- plenty of music;
- heated packs or hot water bottles to comfort you both;
- the best bed and bed linen you can afford;
- a good coffee or tea maker; break-time is crucial;
- scented candles to perfume the air.

CHAPTER 9

Staying Healthy as a Carer

You know what they say during the safety briefings on aeroplanes: in the event that oxygen fails, put your own mask on first before you start trying to help other people.

Sadly, for many carers, our own health comes a long, long way after the health of the person we are caring for. Unlike being in paid work, there's usually no provision for having time off sick – so most carers don't, no matter how ill they are.

Almost two-thirds of carers taking part in the Carers UK 2017 'State of Caring' survey said their physical health had worsened as a result of their caring role: 78 per cent said they were more stressed; 54 per cent said they were able to do less exercise; 45 per cent said they struggled to maintain a balanced diet; and 46 per cent said they'd suffered depression because of their caring role.

But your own health is vital. Vital in order that you can carry on; what will happen if you suddenly collapse? Who would look after your loved one if that happens?

And vital to your own quality of life – and mind – while you're a carer so that you don't end up needing care yourself. However hard-pressed you are, you must make looking after yourself an equal priority to caring for the one you're looking after.

In this chapter we'll look at a few of the health issues that may arise in your carer role.

Carrying out medical procedures

Whether it's doling out tablets or emptying a catheter bag, there may be occasions where caring for someone involves being a nurse, too.

There are several sources for advice. First, you can talk to the professionals; in many cases, the practice or district nurse should be able and willing to give you some training on how to do the things they do at home – after all, you're saving them a job.

If you've time, a first-aid course may be helpful for recognising and dealing with emergencies. St John Ambulance arrange them so ask them what's running in your area. Alternatively, the Red Cross website http://www.redcross.org.uk/What-we-do/First-aid/Everyday-First-Aid has an excellent section on everyday first aid for a wide range of situations, using video and clear instructions on how to respond.

Alternatively you could buy or borrow a first-aid manual. Again, St John Ambulance and the British Red Cross are among those who publish good guides in an easy-to-use format.

The important thing to remember is that if you're not comfortable or confident about giving medical care, you don't have to. You're not a trained nurse and it's perfectly OK to make your feelings clear to the doctor or hospital if you don't want to get involved. They will then make arrangements for a district nurse or doctor to step in.

On the other hand, if you can manage, there'll be less waiting around, fewer clashes with your own routines, and the person you're caring for will know they're in familiar hands.

If they're struggling to take medicines, the most common types are available in a range of forms – not just tablets but capsules, powders, liquids, suppositories, patches, creams or as injections. Ask the doctor if they can try an alternative form.

And while you're at it, ask them to keep you supplied with boxes of surgical gloves and a sharps box if needed. Basic hygiene is important to both of you as someone suffering from one type of health problem may have lower resistance to bugs, and your exhaustion may have the same effect on you.

On that theme, don't worry about appearing rude to anyone who may be harbouring whatever germs are going around; it's common sense to ask them to stay away until they're well again – which means five days symptom free.

Finally, hand washing is crucial – learn how to do the proper NHS hand washing and carry sanitising gel if you're out and about.

Moving and handling

Have I told you the one about taking Mum and her equally disabled friend to a U3A event – in a car with only three doors? Mum still had some movement then, but not enough to prevent her toppling off her seat into the footwell, jammed between the back and front seats. We were certain we'd have to call the fire brigade but luckily a neighbour was passing and between the three of us we somehow managed to prise her out.

Fortunately, other than embarrassment there were no injuries, but we learned our lesson. During the next stage of deterioration, when Mum regularly tripped over her feet and toppled on to the floor, we simply sat with her, keeping her entertained and warm, and waited for the paramedics to arrive with the equipment to get her vertical again.

So really I want to say, 'Don't do it'; it's too risky for them (and for your back). But in the real world there may still be times when you feel you have no choice but to help your loved one up or down or round about.

Make it a last resort, though. There are so many aids that can take the strain and support them getting up from bed, a chair, in and out of the bath, to and from the loo. As we discussed in the last chapter, occupational health should help you with this – and train you in how to use any equipment they bring in.

If you know some tasks are absolutely going to be left to you, then ask the occupational therapist or a health visitor to give you some 'manual handling training' in how to do these things without injuring yourself. Or talk to the nearest carers centre; many of these offer helpful training courses in moving and handling.

Mobility and getting around

Many carers report suffering from cabin fever. Being able to get your loved one out of the house to other activities, even if it's only a nearby park or coffee shop, can be a blessed relief.

Depending on how mobile they are, walking sticks, walking frames and wheeled walkers – with their own seats – can provide stability and a measure of freedom in and outside the house.

Life starts to get a little more complicated with wheelchairs. Disability legislation means there are many more places you can access with a wheelchair and, for those who tire easily, it's increasingly possible to borrow a wheelchair to get around large indoor shopping centres, supermarkets and many visitor attractions such as museums, galleries and stately homes. Just ring ahead to be sure there'll be one available.

Some places, such as dozens of London Underground stations, remain no-go areas. We found public transport the biggest challenge with a wheelchair, closely followed by shops which insist on cramming so many aisles and pop-up displays into the floor space that it's virtually impossible to navigate a route without destroying half the shop.

There is a growing number of disability charities and accessibility campaigners producing really excellent websites and directories that will give you information on access, seating, parking, toilets, wheelchair hire at a host of sites around the UK. See the resources section for a few suggestions.

Of course, there's the Blue Badge scheme, too, for those who quickly give up on the idea that any outing is possible without their own wheels. What you won't know, until the time comes to apply for and use the badge, is that:

- Applying not only involves a tortuous form, but also involves re-applying every three years. It may also involve a personal interview and physical assessment for the person you care for, depending on the local council operating the scheme. It is not for the faint-hearted but, if you are struggling, you can get help with the form from your nearest carers centre or CAB.
- Check first to see if you are automatically eligible; for instance, if you are registered blind or following particular outcomes of the mobility element of your PIP assessment. It will save you time and trouble.
- Once you get your precious Blue Badge, you will discover that there are nothing like enough of the allocated disabled spaces, even though until now it always seemed to you that there were far too many.
- Having a Blue Badge won't automatically exempt you from parking charges. It varies from place to place and car park to car park, so always check what the meter or machine says.
- There are people out there who are not respecters of Blue Badge

spaces. These are people who have never been carers, or disabled themselves. Their time will come . . .

The taboo of incontinence

'When we cleared Mum's house, it was heartbreaking to find stained pants stuffed to the back of the wardrobe. She'd obviously been incontinent for a while but been too embarrassed to get help. After she came to live with us, it was the thing she found hardest, needing me to clean her up after another accident. She used to say, "I never thought it would come to this."'

Bev

I've taken my time getting to this most horrible of the health challenges you may face. Because it's usually equally awful and undignified for them and for you.

Though most parents take a matter-of-fact approach to mopping up their children's accidents, loss of bladder or bowel control in adults is complicated by its associations with lack of personal hygiene, loss of control and of dignity.

Having waged a daily war against the sharp smell of urine, and more than once been forced to use a mop and bucket on the pavement outside Mum's house after an explosive episode, I no longer find any comedian's casual jokes about incontinence the slightest bit funny.

And yet, ironically, allowing ourselves to see the funny side and make a joke of it with our loved ones may be the best way of coping with something so difficult that until it happens to someone you care about you'll find it's hardly ever discussed.

If incontinence becomes a problem, the first thing to do is check whether there is a medical cause and therefore medical help available. Speak to your loved one's doctor or district nurse who can bring in the continence nurse to do an assessment and offer advice and practical support. Sometimes particular drugs or combinations of medicines can cause loss of control, and diet or an infection may also be a factor.

If medical problems are ruled out the next step is to see if you can set up routines that will minimise the chances of accidents happening. Get the person you care for in the habit of going to the loo at set times; ensure the loo – or at least a commode or bottles or bedpan – are close by; and ensure they don't have a lot to drink just before bed.

If incontinence has become a fact of life, the continence nurse will be able to advise on the most suitable products to minimise the impact on you both, and they should also be able to arrange a supply of pads or pants free of charge. If not, or if the supply never lasts as long as the month, they're stocked by all big chemists. As they're bulky items, many companies offer a home delivery service. There are also agencies who will collect soiled items and clean up. The continence adviser should be able to give you details.

Waterproof bedding beneath the sheets will offer some protection, as will cleanable surfaces such as lino or laminate in preference to carpet on the floor. Clothes that give quick and easy access will also help. And more sophisticated aids coming on the market now include a loo which squirts water up to clean soiled areas.

But remember, if you're really struggling, your caring role does not have to include what is coyly known as 'personal care'. You can tell social services you don't want to be involved and those tasks will have to be taken over by paid carers. Age UK offers a free booklet on managing incontinence, *Bladder and Bowel Problems*, available by post or directly downloadable from its website.

Self-care

So that's them; how are we going to keep you healthy when you've already told all those surveys you don't have time for exercise or healthy eating, and your mental health is sometimes fragile?

How about a few short suggestions along the lines of 'If you only have time to take care of your health a little, then at least do a few of these things'?

High-speed health tips

- No time or money for a gym membership? Take a ten-minute walk around the block every day if you can. Don't under-estimate the power of a short walk, change of scene and fresh air to clear away staleness and restore a little peace to your over-busy mind. Walking is one of the kindest things you can do for you.
- If you're too tired to walk or don't have the energy, then looking at something green – a tree, a field, a bit of parkland, a plant in the garden – can have similar benefits. It works better if there is no glass between you and whatever it is you choose to focus on.
- As for that endlessly busy mind, start to meditate. There's no secret to it but the benefits are enormous and recognised by just about every health expert, especially for children and young people. There are dozens of phone apps to help – Headspace, Calm and Insight Timer are my favourites. If your caring doesn't even allow you ten minutes' escape into a calming meditation, then why not suggest you both listen to a little 'music' in silence.
- Eat well. If you can't find time to cook then healthy snacks such as nuts, fruit, cheese and oatcakes are miles better than crisps and doughnuts. Always have a supply with you to deal with energy dips. And whenever someone asks how they can help you, then suggest they cook and freeze one portion of whatever they're cooking for themselves for you each week.

- Take breaks. Whatever you think, you cannot do it all. Whether you're caring full-time or rushing between responsibilities at home, work and your loved one, you must schedule in time out for you. And by the way, I'm going to keep repeating this until I see you doing it.

More food for thought

A good and balanced diet is important for you both, but a challenge to provide if there already aren't enough hours in the day. Rather than planning big meals two or three times a day, you might find it easier to have snack stops: sandwiches, fruit, cheese and biscuits, milk shakes, soup, cereals. It's also a way of breaking up the hours if time weighs heavily on the hands of the person you care for.

For those unable to prepare or even heat their own food, meals-on-wheels services are still available, usually contracted out to private suppliers. Social services will be able to tell you who to contact. For the slightly more mobile, social services can also advise on the many suppliers of frozen pre-prepared meals operating a home-delivery service. One advantage is that their menus these days are wide and cater for all types of diets, which means the person you're caring for gets more choice about what they want to eat.

If you're living on a diet of ready meals, do think about taking dietary supplements, for instance an A-Z multivitamin/mineral every day. How many of us genuinely have enough time to check that we're getting enough selenium and magnesium and, as the doctor says, 'It won't do you any harm – and it might do you a lot of good.' Some of these are also available in energy or dietary drinks – expensive but a quick and pleasant way of keeping your system topped up with essentials.

And I mentioned asking friends, neighbours or relatives to help keep your freezer stocked. You may want to do the same for yourself –

doubling portions every time you cook, then freezing one lot for those days when the only thing you're capable of is flopping in the chair.

Fit for life

You may never have been a great fan of exercise, but even if you think that pilates is a rather unpleasant medical condition, now you're a carer the way to look at exercise is as 'time out'.

Don't be fooled into convincing yourself all that running around, up and down stairs, between home and work, to the shops and appointments, is keeping you fit – activity under stress is almost worse than no activity at all. Your body is wound like a spring and liable to snap.

The best thing about 'formal' exercise is that it has a positive effect on your mind as well as your body. Methods such as yoga or tai chi actually train your mind to be still for a while, at the same time as your body is being gently stretched. Even a hectic game of squash, badminton or other competitive sport has a relaxing effect on both body and mind because it requires concentration. And thinking about the game temporarily squeezes out the million other things that concern you as a carer.

If you're one of the, er … 100 per cent … of carers who feel guilty taking time out, then why not sign up for some kind of sponsored activity? You may feel less guilty about the training if the goal is to raise funds to support other carers, or people suffering from the same condition as your loved one.

And if the only way you can get out is by taking the person you care for with you – and their health allows it – then do so. Find out whether the local leisure centres run any special exercise classes you can both join. Or investigate what your local Age UK or carers centre has on offer.

Mind your mind

As a carer your mind is active a lot of the time – in the middle of the night when you should be sleeping, in the bath when you're attempting to relax, or throughout the day, churning relentlessly on to what you've got to do next before you're halfway through the task in hand. Unfortunately, that's not the kind of brain food that acts as a stimulant to feeling good.

And then there's the person you're caring for. If they are often confined to the home, cut off by circumstances from regular contact with friends and other family, time will move as achingly slowly for them as it hurtles by for you. What you both need is to give your mind a regular workout with an activity you enjoy, the kind of occupations that require so much concentration you simply can't think about anything else.

Below are a few activities that other carers recommend for you to try together or apart:

- join a craft group;
- get a tape recorder and record your loved one's story; then record your own;
- read aloud to each other, or borrow books on tape;
- go to the cinema once a week or once a month and take it in turns to choose what you watch. If you can't get out, recreate the movies at home by making popcorn and pulling the curtains;
- try one of the huge selection of mindful colouring books available from your local bookstore;
- invent a recipe for a satisfying soup or a delicious dessert;
- attend a lecture at the local college or the nearest U3A;
- visit any special exhibitions that come to your local art gallery or museum;
- learn to identify the birds and other wildlife that visit the garden; and learn how to attract more.

- join a book group – online if you can't get out – or start your own;
- sign up for an adult education class;
- do a distance learning course in anything from languages to creative writing at home;
- join a carers support group!

We'll return to the subject of your health and well-being in a few chapters. I warned you I wouldn't let it drop!

CHAPTER 10

Warning: Rocky Relationships Ahead

When author Sue Miller got a phone call to say the police had picked up her father wandering confused through a strange town, her biggest challenge was how to shift her thinking – to recognise that the man who'd always looked out for her now needed her to be strong for him.

In a moving account of her father's Alzheimer's, *The Story of My Father,* Sue describes the moment their relationship changed: 'It became clear to me that I would need to be honest and forceful or he would never accede to me. That I would need to insist. I had never insisted on anything with my father . . . (but) *we would be in charge of him now.'*

Husbands and wives who suddenly find themselves caring for a partner also speak of their struggle to adjust, sometimes overnight, to a dramatically altered relationship. Whatever vows they may have made, neither had ever seriously considered the possibility that a major accident or illness would force one of them into the role of total dependent, the other into being their carer.

Parents, too, have perhaps spent two decades nurturing their children and look forward to getting a little more of their lives back. Then they find that severe mental illness, drug or alcohol dependency makes it impossible to loosen the ties of care. Their responsibilities now seem to stretch for ever into the future.

And then there are the relationships with other family members; perhaps they want to be supportive but can't help minding sometimes that so much of you is now focused on your caring role.

We're often told we have to work at relationships, but what happens when you have neither the time nor energy for yet more 'work'?

Along with all the other issues caring throws up, its effects on our relationships with those we are caring for, and those around us, are among the most profound. What can you do to help yourself and others face up to them and move forward in your altered world?

In this chapter, we'll look at some of the challenges of changing relationships and what you can do to ensure your relationships remain a source of love and support rather than difficulty and distrust.

Becoming a parent to your parent

> *'I think the worst thing for me was that Mum and I never got on when I was a kid. It was always my brother this, my brother that, and I resented it. I thought, "Why should I have to look after you? You hated me when I was a kid and now I'm lumbered."'*

Linda

As the parents among you know, our children remain our children no matter how old they get. Even when they have children of their own, we're still looking out for them.

Conversely, as adults many of us remain children around our parents, hanging on to the same patterns of behaviour, still looking to them for approval, recognition and support.

Whether you get on with your parents or not, the deep familiarity of this first, key relationship is what makes it so challenging to relate as carer and cared-for, to make decisions, take over the finances, or look after the physical needs of someone who used to do so for you.

Of course, there are also carers like Linda who never experienced a sense of being looked after by their parents, which brings its own set of special difficulties when the roles seem to be reversed.

Along with all this, it's likely you will be dealing with your parent's mixed feelings about being in this situation at all; worry about being 'a burden', frustration which translates into being cantankerous with you, denial, or insistence on continuing to treat you like a child.

Whether you grew up in a loving home or a very challenging one, it may help to remind yourself that some of the difficulties in your relationship probably existed before you became carer and cared-for. The dramatic change in how you relate, plus the amount of time you now spend together, will have brought existing tensions into sharper focus. But perhaps it's also a chance to go a little way towards healing them?

Do seek help from a counsellor or carers centre if you feel the issues are difficult enough to be getting in the way of your carer role, or causing either of you real grief.

Continue to be child and parent

This is a difficult one – especially if, like Sue Miller, your parent has a condition that makes them incapable of making the best choices for themselves. You want to keep them healthy and safe and that will mean making decisions for them and about them rather than *with* them.

But even in such cases I'd advise that, for both your sakes, you resist a complete role reversal for as long as you can. One of the pitfalls of treating your loved one as a child is that they may become more dependent. Think back to when you were a child, or to your own children. The more people did for you, the less inclined you were to do things like picking up your own clothes or making your bed yourself. At whatever level your parent is able to operate, be clear with them about their responsibilities.

Health and social services operate under the terms of the Mental Capacity Act 2005 which says a person is presumed to have capacity unless they have had an assessment showing that they don't – even if the decisions they make are not necessarily wise or the choices you'd make for them.

Mum's character changed in countless ways after her stroke; one small change was that she suddenly developed a taste for venison and best steak whereas before she'd lived on mince and mashed potato. My sister and I talked about where we needed to draw the line between protecting her from going broke and recognising that at a time when illness had robbed her of so much, her diet and buying treats for herself were areas where she could still exercise choice. So, mostly, we zipped our lips and got out the frying pan.

If your parent is in a similar position, think about which areas of their life you can encourage them to continue to make choices about.

Some carers say it's helped their relationship if they are able to find opportunities for their parents to continue to parent them, for instance seeking their advice, whether on an important life choice or how get a Yorkshire pudding to rise. Just because you are having to dress or bathe them, it doesn't mean they don't still have something to contribute in other areas of life. As another carer, Bill, says, 'I've been looking after my father's physical needs for some time now and I can see it bothers him that I have to do it. So I've started to talk to him about some of my problems, things going on in my life and given him a chance to offer his take on them. Not only is his advice often spot on, it makes him feel we have a more equal relationship. He's still my dad.'

Increasingly, we've discovered that music memories are some of the last to go; some people can recall songs and sing them when they can't recall anything else. The same may be true of scents and smells so think about the ways in which you *can* still connect with your loved one through such memories, and connect them with *their* past.

You could also experiment with ways of reinventing your relationship. After her father's diagnosis, Sue Miller recounts how much pleasure it gave her to organise for him the same kind of treats she'd enjoyed as a child – a drive out, sandwiches on a park bench, an ice cream on the way home, both of their faces alight with the joy of rediscovering sights, sounds and experiences they thought they'd left behind.

Hers is a lovely example of how, sometimes, becoming a carer to your parent can change the relationship in positive ways. A parent who has always been distant or disapproving is now vulnerable, and your feelings towards them soften as their hardness is replaced with gratitude for your care.

Caring for a partner

Lesley and John looked to have it sussed. They'd brought up two lovely children and in their forties gave up high-pressured jobs to run a bookshop together. They were sociable, loyal to their friends, and obviously still in love after all these years.

One night a friend who hadn't seen them for a while got a call out of the blue from Lesley. She sounded odd and confused. John called the same friend the next day to explain Lesley had just been diagnosed as having early onset dementia. He said, 'I feel better knowing what's wrong. I couldn't understand the way she'd been recently. But I'm scared. I'm just beginning to realise that all these years she's always been the one looking after me, taking care of everything. I don't know if I'll cope.'

For one partner to become dependent on the other is to shift a marriage or loving partnership on its axis. The very term 'partnership' conjures up equals, sharing, dreaming, building together and yet suddenly that has changed. On top of dealing with day-to-day care, you may be having to come to terms with the loss of the future you had planned, with the loss of your best friend, a sexual companion, a co-parent.

The same may be true for them, of course, as well as the gamut of emotions they may be running about their changed circumstances, their need to be dependent on you, and perhaps their fears about its impact on you, too.

This is a huge amount of loss and emotion to contemplate and will need time, care and honest and loving conversation to work a way through. Most of us aren't in perfect relationships so do think about seeking professional support with what is happening, either for yourself alone or as a couple. Relate are still the relationship experts but your local carers centre may also offer counselling services.

Depending on your partner's condition, a trained counsellor will be able to work with you both to find out what you can still be to each other, despite your changed circumstances.

If your relationship was a very long way short of perfect, and has been for some time, you may suddenly find yourself feeling 'saddled'. Before your partner became ill, you'd sometimes considered ending the relationship; now they're dependent on you, you no longer feel you have any choice but to stay. What would people think if you choose not to?

There are no hard and fast rules about what you should do, as Kim discovered. 'The twenty-year age gap between us was never a problem until he developed a serious heart condition. Suddenly here I am wanting to do so many things with my life but he's an old man. I just can't be his carer. I know how that sounds to other people but I've done it before for my dad and I can't do it again. I won't leave him but I've accepted a job that takes me away from home during the week. While I'm away, he has paid carers coming in to look after him.'

Just remember that no matter what other people think, if something doesn't work for you and is making you unhappy, then it is unlikely to work well for anyone else.

Let's talk about sex

In *The Selfish Pig's Guide to Caring*, Hugh Marriott describes the effect being a carer has on our sex lives as one of the great unspoken secrets. So many of us come at sex through our feelings; if those change, our need or desire for sex will be altered, too.

Having to perform intimate tasks for your partner may well affect the way you feel about them, especially if there are times when you feel more like a parent or brother or sister to them. Sexual desire may start to feel inappropriate, even distasteful. Or it may be that dealing with all the other emotions caring brings up, as well as its physical demands, simply leaves you no energy to want sex.

Your feelings are perfectly reasonable and you need to respect them. But that may be easier said than done if the person you're caring for still wants a sexual relationship with you. Their condition may not have affected their sex drive; indeed, it may have heightened it. At the same time, their feelings of dependency may lead them to see sex as a way of reassuring themselves that you continue to love them.

Here again, you should seek help from a relationship counsellor, who may refer you to a psychosexual counsellor. They are trained to help you look at such difficult feelings in a safe environment and will be neither judgemental nor shocked. They'll have encountered people who feel the way you do many times before, help you work out if there are ways of meeting some of your and your partner's needs, and assist you to live with the feelings you have.

And then there is the possibility that though *you've* lost sexual feeling for your partner, you haven't lost desire altogether. Particularly if you are still relatively young when you become your partner's carer, the fear that you may have to live for years or even the rest of your life without sex can add considerably to the stress you are already under.

Only you know how you feel about the notion of finding other ways to have your sexual needs met. Your religious views may prohibit you seeking sexual relations outside of your marriage – and so might your timetable! But if sex is important to you then you need to recognise that it contributes significantly to your physical and emotional well-being. And since you cannot be the best carer you can be if your own needs are being denied, then your usual notions of what is appropriate behaviour may no longer fit in this new world you find yourself in.

Communication is key

In all of these changing relationships, don't overlook the fact that – if you are still able to have meaningful conversations – time spent talking with your loved one about their expectations and wishes can be quite revealing. They may not want you to do what you want to do for them. Or they may want or expect more from you. Honest conversations are vital with the person needing help.

Sometimes, we avoid them out of fear that they may only add to our burden, when in fact, the opposite can be true. The person needing help may well have been a carer at some time in their life and knows all too well the stresses and strains of this. Some may take the line that it is pay-back now they need care, but most will shy away from placing that burden on their family. Talking about this can help the relationship and improve understanding between carer and cared-for.

Children who remain dependent

One hurdle you may face as a parent carer is knowing how and when to give your child more independence, to allow them to develop as far as they are able and perhaps leave the family home.

Mary says it was isolation and lack of support that prevented her from seeing this until it was almost too late. The result of what she describes as 'being cocooned together for years' was that her daughter finally became violent. 'We were just stifling each other. She didn't have anywhere to go like other teenagers and say, "My mum's doing my head in." When I started getting bruises, I called social services.'

Her daughter is now in a supported living setting but the traumatic way they parted means both continue to find the letting-go hard. 'The first three weeks she must have phoned me eighty times which was really wearing. Finally, I realised if I ran to her every time we'd end up back at square one.'

As a parent carer, it's important to recognise that you will still have to go through all the same struggles and stages as any other parent and child. In any family, the relationship between parent and child changes often and you need to let that happen and not confuse the difficulties of providing care with the usual ups, downs and growing pains every parent-child relationship encounters.

If you're struggling, do consult other carers, especially those you may meet through support groups set up specifically by and for the parents of others whose children suffer from the same illness or disability. They can help you navigate the road that leads to more independence for you both.

To add to the challenges of transition, carers have found some local authorities are better than others at managing whatever comes after school for your child. It's not unknown for the local authority to assume you, the child's parent, are sorting out post-school provision – further education, training, residential care – yourself. If your child is approaching adulthood and no one has mentioned plans for the future, get on to them and insist you get together to discuss who is going to do what to ensure your child doesn't fall through a gap.

Returning to the nest

And what of those children who need to return home because of illness or disability that develops later in life?

Pete and Sarah were already retired when it became clear that their adult daughter's mental-health issues meant she couldn't manage alone. Rather than see her move to a secure unit, they chose to have her home. But they were already struggling with their own health issues and say that each day they feel as if they are living on a knife edge, wondering if today is the day they will walk into their daughter's bedroom and find she's succeeded in taking her own life. 'We did what we felt was best. What parent wouldn't? But if we had our time again, we wouldn't do it. We have no lives now; nothing but worrying about her. And then what happens when we go?' Pete admits.

It's entirely normal to step up when your children need you but if your knee-jerk reaction is to become your adult child's carer, do take time to consider the following questions first:

- What impact will this have on your own life and health?
- What about your other relationships, particularly with siblings?
- In what setting will your adult child get the best support?
- Do they need the company of their own age group?
- If you have them at home, are there facilities they can go to in the day to give you some space and time?

Once again, your local carers centre and talking to other carers may help you make the best choice for everyone. Which is not to say that it will be the perfect choice. This is a good moment to say out loud that just as there are rarely perfect relationships, so there are almost never perfect choices. 'Good enough' may have to do, even if that means feeling guilty.

We'll look at carers and guilt in a later chapter.

Family matters

'Despite the expense of buying a house that's larger than you needed, despite the money involved in creating an annex, despite the security you've created and the safety you've offered, you'll still never be the favourite son or daughter. Far from it. You'll hear constant news of how well your useless siblings are doing and what good children they are, despite the fact that they've drained your elderly relative's finances and buggered off to New Zealand to avoid any responsibility. (I know this makes me sound bitter and twisted – but I am).'

Anonymous contributor to Age Space:
www.agespace.org/10-things-no-one-tells-you

One of the saddest things about becoming carer to her mother was that it estranged Lizzie from her sister Anne. When their mother could no longer cope with living alone, it was Lizzie who was the nearest. Rather than move her into residential care, Lizzie decided she'd sell her own house and move in with their mother so she could support her in familiar surroundings.

Lizzie says, 'Anne and I spoke about it and I thought she was OK with the decision. It turns out she wasn't. She thought I was trying to get hold of Mum's money and property for myself. That hurt me more than anything because, as far as I was concerned, I'd put my life on hold to help Mum. Anne never lifted a finger, not really. Perhaps I should have told her I was feeling dumped on by her and she might have been able to be honest about her worries. We haven't spoken since Mum died.'

Lizzie and Anne's broken relationship is a salutary lesson in the importance of frequent and honest communication among all those who have a stake in your caring role.

It may seem unfair that as well as being a carer you're having to make the running in talking to other relatives – as if you don't have enough to do. There are certainly plenty of cases where carers feel, quite rightly, that other family members aren't doing enough; that they have literally been left 'holding the baby' because they live nearest, or aren't working, or have fewer responsibilities.

On the other hand, those same relatives may say they feel 'squeezed out'. That you're so busy taking care of your loved one there's no longer a role for them. At the risk of wading into the minefield of family relationships, it's important to recognise that few of us really see things the way they are.

Rather, we experience the world through the filter of our beliefs and experience. We tell ourselves stories about what is going on based on past experience and on beliefs – such as 'If I don't sort this out no one else will.' These beliefs may or may not bear any relation to the truth.

The only way to know what is going on is for them and you to talk and listen in equal measure to each other. It's possible other family members might want to do more but feel shut out by the closeness of your relationship with their loved one. Maybe there are times when, without realising it, you make it hard for them to get involved because keeping control is your way of coping. Maybe the fact that you've never involved them in any decision-making has triggered old beliefs, jealousies or suspicions in them.

An effective way of stepping outside the situation that's causing you difficulty is to try out this exercise, doing what the native Americans call 'walking a mile in their moccasins'.

Change Your Perspective, Change Your Relationships

Even when people seem to be behaving badly or being deliberately difficult, it helps to take a step away from our own reaction to them in order to understand what need, thought or belief lies behind their behaviour. This simple exercise helps you to do that:

1. Close your eyes and think of somebody you are having a problem with. Imagine that person is standing in front of you now. As clearly as you can, notice what you are thinking and feeling, hear any thoughts in your head or words you spoke to them. Then, picture yourself drifting up from your own body and down into theirs.

2. Now you're in the shoes of the person you struggle with, looking back at yourself. For a moment, see how the world looks from their perspective. What is going on in their head? What are they feeling? What lies behind their words and those feelings? What are they saying to themselves about the situation? Now, once again, drift up from their body and into that of a third person, someone outside the situation whose intelligence and wisdom you admire.

3. Step into their shoes and imagine them watching the two of you interact. How do they see the situation as a neutral observer? What are they seeing as they watch you? Do they have any insights to share?

4. Finally, move back into your own shoes. Take what you have learned and look at the person you are having problems with in a new way. What do you now want to say or do to move the relationship forward or take a step towards some resolution of your problems?

All of that said, if they genuinely aren't pulling their weight then you are absolutely entitled to tell them so, find out why and ask for more help. Take another look at the section in this book on assertiveness (in Chapter 4), which should help you be honest and clear with your relatives without anger or other negative feelings getting in the way. And have a long and honest think about the items in the checklist below which may be affecting all of your relationships.

Everyone around you has a stake in how you being a carer will affect your relationships, so the following tips are worth considering:

- Share as much of the practical care as you can. It's a way of reinforcing that you are a family and all members have responsibility for each other.
- Are you sure you're not excluding them? When we're under pressure we often feel it's quicker and easier to do things ourselves. Ask them if they ever feel as if you're cutting them out.
- Organise regular family meetings to keep everyone in touch. If geography prevents you physically getting together, organise an online family conference through an online communication tool such as Zoom.
- Recognise that other people make different choices and you can't change them. Your siblings, friends or family may be well aware of what you are doing as a carer but choose not to get involved. If you don't let go of your expectations of them, your feelings of resentment will hurt you more than them.

- Be aware that family issues, roles and resentments from the past may be revived by this new, stressful situation. Try to avoid getting 'hooked in' to the past.
- Don't try and be a counsellor for everyone. As the main carer, you may feel pressured by others into acting as a counsellor for them. But you can't take on everyone's problems – and they shouldn't expect you to.
- Don't be defined by your carer role. You are so much more.

How caring can affect those closest to home

'I mostly feel like I'm walking on eggshells – I'm so mindful that any request of time (even for something fun or pleasant) could become a burden. Over the years, I have definitely learned to hold back from asking.'

Amy

Inevitably, if one member of the family requires more from you, others (including you) will end up with less. There are only twenty-four hours in a day – even in a carer's day. You may not be in a position to do much about this, but being aware of it and acknowledging it is important for everyone.

For instance, don't assume that other family members, especially children, will just naturally understand why they can't have more of your time and attention. Understand their jealousy or resentment if that's what they are feeling and remind them and yourself that those feelings are pretty normal in households without any illness or disability. Every child wants to be the centre of his or her parent's life. Regular check-in time will give them a chance to express what they are feeling; this really is a case where the quality of the time you are able to give them is worth more than its quantity.

At the same time, watch yourself for any signs that you are leaning on them more than you should be, making them *your* carers. There is a big difference between asking them to do their fair share of chores, contributing to the household, and looking to them for emotional support. However much of a carer you are, you remain their parent and should be looking to other adults for the support you need.

If you live with a partner, that relationship is going to need your attention, too. It may be that you're never in the same room because you're taking it in turns to care. Or because you are carrying the load as a carer while practicalities such as the need for an income or to care for others in the house mean your partner is always fully occupied with their duties. You're like trains on parallel tracks, watching each other hurtle along at speed but never close enough or slow enough to make meaningful contact.

Adversity can sometimes bring people closer together. For every carer who regrets the way a marriage, civil partnership or special relationship was damaged by the amount of energy they had to put into someone else, there is another for whom their partner proved an anchor, the solidity at the core of their lives.

The thing to keep reminding yourself is that while the day-to-day health of your relationship may be affected by your carer role, its strength depends on precisely the same things as any other loving relationship, including all those in which no one is a carer – your commitment to each other and to making it work, to sharing yourselves and your feelings, to being honest with each other, and to supporting and being supported by each other.

Sandwich carers

I'm probably typical of this new so-called "sandwich generation"... I'm 50ish, have three school-age children, a husband who is often away from home with work, my own business and three relatives in their eighties who need varying and increasing amounts of my time and attention. It's not uncommon for me to go straight from the school run to a doctor's appointment with my mother, or to my aunt's care home, while also taking work calls. It's a slightly different version of "having it all", and though there are days when I feel glad to be able to juggle these responsibilities and be there for the people in my life who matter most, I can't pretend there aren't other days when I find it all overwhelming.'

Ruth

According to Carers UK, we are in the middle of a new social phenomenon – the 'sandwich generation'. The expression usually refers to those looking after school-age children at the same time as caring for older parents. But today's complex family relationships can lead to people having a variety of multiple caring responsibilities for people in different generations.

Research by the Centre for Longitudinal Studies (*Caring Responsibilities in Middle Age*, 2014) concluded that the so-called sandwich generation is becoming one of the 'hardest pressed generations'.

Increased awareness of this may not yet have led to the sort of investment that sandwich carers need in order to be able to cope with the demands of being stuck in the middle. But if you are a sandwich carer, you may get a smidgen of comfort from recognising that you are part of a phenomenon that policymakers will eventually *have* to pay more attention to.

It's not all bad

I've written a lot about the challenges to all kinds of relationships and hope some of the ideas and tools may help you navigate such tricky waters. However, it wouldn't be fair to leave you with the impression that every relationship will suffer because you are a carer.

One of the gifts of our mum's illness and disability is that it's brought my sister and me even closer together. We've always been best friends but her decision to move geographically closer to help care for Mum means what she calls 'Team Matthews' is more solid than ever.

We've learned we must consciously remember to talk to each other about the rest of our lives, rather than always getting bogged down in practicalities about Mum's care. And we've become ruthless about insisting the other takes breaks. As I said, we all need to remind ourselves not to be defined by our role as carers.

Then there's Mum herself. I won't pretend she and I had an easy relationship for the first five decades of my life. It was as messy and conflicted as some of your relationships are likely to be. But with the stroke came a softening in both of us that means when her time comes to go, I will have less baggage to deal with than I might otherwise have done. I know I've done my best.

I'm lucky in this sense, I know. Just as I'm lucky to be a part of a small but very close and supportive family who have rallied round with help and endless understanding whenever they're able.

A friend of mine was completely estranged from her father. Then she got a text telling her that he had a terminal illness and didn't want to see her. She ignored the text and insisted on travelling to see him, working with him to understand his needs and supporting him in his last months. In consequence of her care, she's found it much easier to be reconciled to his memory.

You may or may not be as fortunate – but it is worth looking around at your relationships and seeing if there is indeed anything you can find to be grateful for. It won't change your situation but choosing to focus, if only for a few minutes, on where the glass is half full rather than half empty, will make *you* feel better. And that's what I care about.

CHAPTER 11

Some Guidance for Young Carers

We've just been looking at how relationships can be altered by our caring role. That is never more true than for the estimated 700,000 young people who currently find themselves responsible as carers for *their* parent or parents – one in twelve of all secondary school-age children, according to Carers Trust.

For young people, being a carer for an adult could involve anything from helping out with practical tasks such as housework and shopping to helping them get out of bed or take their medicines. If you are under eighteen or a young adult reading this, perhaps you give up your free time to help care for your brothers and sisters. Perhaps you help a parent or other adult manage their money, or communicate with others. Or perhaps a family member or friend sees you as the shoulder they can lean on whenever they are distressed or not coping with their life. Maybe you're living with a single parent and have stepped into the gap left by the missing adult – so that sometimes you feel as if you are more of a partner to your parent than a child.

Like every other carer, your life may have started to revolve around someone else's needs for any number of reasons. Because the person you care for became ill or is disabled, or because their problems – for instance, some kind of dependency or mental-health problem – prevent them caring fully for you and your brothers and sisters.

You may feel that you were given no choice; that your life just is the way it is.

But it's so important that you know you *do* have choices and there are other adults and organisations standing by to support you.

It's natural to worry about your parent, and to want to protect them. But it should not be left to you to look after them alone. If you haven't yet done so, please tell someone at school. Carers Trust found 68 per cent of young carers had experienced bullying at school but only half had someone at school supporting them. Teachers don't always know what's going on in our lives unless we tell them, and it's important you have someone to turn to at a place you spend so much of your time.

It's also worthwhile thinking about who else you might trust with what's going on for you – your feelings, your fears and concerns. Perhaps it could be the parent of one of your friends, another relative or family friend, or someone else in your local community?

You are showing, just by being a carer, how responsible you are, but there is help out there that other adults can help you access.

Get in touch with a carers centre

Carers centres throughout the UK offer special services to young carers like you, including putting you in touch with other young carers who will understand what you're going through in a way no one else can.

You can find out if there's one close to you by visiting https://carers. org/our-work-locally and entering your postcode. If you're a long way from the nearest centre, you can still talk in confidence to other young carers online. Carers UK runs a forum and Childline a message board for young carers.

Young carers have rights

This brings me to your rights as a young carer. It may seem strange that you have the right *not* to feel anxious or scared because of your caring role. Most of us can remember how, as children, the things that worried or frightened us seemed so huge. But for you as a young carer, those could be feelings, along with sadness or loneliness, that you have every day.

You also have the right *not* to be doing a caring role that affects your health or your friendships, your school or college work or your plans for your own future.

To help you try and keep your own life on track, the law expects your local council to come in and find out what your life is like, what your caring role involves, what you want and what support you need in order to have the same opportunites as other people your age. This is called a 'young carer's needs assessment' and the sort of questions you'll be asked and what information the council wants to know will depend on your age. But here are a few ideas that you might want to make notes on; we all find it difficult sometimes to remember everything we meant to say.

- What are the things you do to help around the house – this could be every day or just once in a while?
- What are the things you do to help the person you are supporting – again, this could be every day or now and then?
- How do you think helping this person affects *your* life – your schooling, your friendships, your free time?
- What about your feelings? How do you feel day to day? Are you struggling with anything?
- Are there any people helping or listening to *you?*

- What are the things you'd like to do that you can't because you're looking after this family member or friend?
- Do you have any ideas about what would help you?

Getting an assessment

In a perfect world, someone will see that you're a young carer and make sure you get this assessment. I hope that happens. But if it hasn't, then I really hope you can think of another adult who will contact the council for you and start the ball rolling.

If not, you are entitled to contact the council yourself and ask for an assessment. Or go to the back of this book and find the details for one of the organisations for young people who can tell you what to do.

A charter for young carers

Other young people in your position have come up with their own charter, setting out what we, as adults, owe to you:

Young Carers' Charter
Children and young people have the right to:

- **be children as well as carers**
- **get support from school and college to ensure a good education**
- **have time from caring for friendship, fun and to pursue other interests**
- **have help and support so they are not caring alone**
- **be listened to**
- **be safe**
- **have a break**

- **be involved and given information by the other people and agencies that are involved**
- **be able to stop caring when they need to**
- **be helped to move on into adult life**

A final word on watching out for young carers: if you're reading this as an adult carer, it's worth just mentioning that there may be invisible young carers in your own life. We don't always see what's right under our noses.

Does your work, do your spare-time interests or family time bring you into contact with any of these young people who, like you, may not have recognised there's a name for what they do, as well as rights and needs?

We've already agreed you have a lot on your plate keeping yourself going sometimes, but a simple call to your nearest carers centre, or to your local council, may set in train the help that will transform the loneliness, confusion and struggle that so many young carers experience.

Just like you, in fact.

CHAPTER 12

So, How Are You Feeling?

'Nobody cares for me. I feel as if I'm in a Hollywood film and do not exist except as a support character and somebody else is always in the starring role. I have more in common with the stairlift than people – relied upon and only noticed if I break down.'

Penny

One of the toughest things about caring for my uncle was knowing what to do with some of the things I was feeling: resentment at being left alone to care for him; anger that he assumed my time was his and would continue to be; frustration that my plans for life were on hold; fear that this would go on for ever; guilt, that I felt all these things when it was him who was dying.

And, believe me, those feelings were only the tip of a very substantial iceberg.

No matter what your motivations for being a carer, what circumstances brought you to this point, it's likely that as well as dealing with daily life you are having to cope with a whole range of difficult feelings. It's also quite likely that your way of coping is by pretending those feelings aren't even there, or suppressing them because:

- You're ashamed of them – you must be a 'bad person' to feel the way you do when it's your loved one who is suffering.
- You're scared that owning your feelings may be like opening Pandora's box – if you allow yourself to feel as you do, all those pent-up emotions may just swamp and overwhelm you and who knows what would happen then to your ability to carry on?
- You think they're a sign of weakness – if you could toughen up, be a better person or love the person you care for more, then you wouldn't be feeling this way.
- Feelings? What are they? You were brought up in the school of the stiff upper lip and told off if you ever became loud or angry or resentful.

The thing is, our feelings are like warning lights on a car dashboard. They start flashing precisely *because* there is something wrong that we need to pay attention to. You wouldn't ignore those warning lights in your car, would you, knowing that to do so would almost certainly lead to a break down?

The so-called 'curse of the strong' is to do the same when it comes to our feelings, putting up with and shutting up instead of allowing ourselves to recognise what we're feeling and deal with those emotions in healthy ways.

Consider this. There are more than 150 carers support groups throughout the UK – and those groups only exist because so many carers need someone to support them. No matter how unacceptable some of those emotions are to you, there are hundreds of thousands of others who actually *do* know how you feel – because they feel the same way sometimes.

That's what this chapter is about: helping you to recognise what you're feeling when you're feeling it, know when you may need to respond, and understand how you can do so effectively – without anyone getting hurt.

Feel those feelings

Before we look at some of the emotions many of us experience as carers, a word about getting in touch with your feelings. A moment ago I mentioned the stiff upper lip. That's one way some us learned how (not) to deal with our feelings. Or the reverse may be true – you grew up in a home where there was *too* much feeling going on. Perhaps one of the adults was angry – even violent – and you learned that emotion could be dangerous.

As for fear, when you were frightened were your feelings acknowledged, or were you brusquely told, 'There's nothing to be scared of!'?

It's not our parents' fault. They couldn't teach us what *they* hadn't been taught, but it is useful to recognise that many of us do not grow up getting help, or seeing good examples, of how to deal with difficult feelings.

Putting the lid on them may allow us to function for a while, but if your caring role goes on and on, if it continues to get harder, one of two things may happen:

1. Your bottled-up emotions eventually overflow and start to seep out wherever they can. You get furious with the people you love best or, conversely, with complete strangers, queues in the shops and traffic jams. You find yourself furious behind the wheel or rushing angrily at everything. In other words, someone is going to get hurt.

2. Your own mental health suffers because when you lock down the difficult feelings you are also locking down the ones that make life worth living: love, joy, gratitude, peace. It's not possible to tell our minds to allow some feelings but not others, which can lead to a sense of flatlining. Or even, if it goes on too long, depression or burnout.

How to feel, express and release your feelings

Let me say again, we're not wrong for having the feelings that we do. They're a normal part of human experience. The thing to do with feelings is to discharge them safely. Only then is it safe for us to consider whether there is anything else we need do, like speak out or make changes.

Try this simple exercise when you're feeling emotional; better still, get in the habit of doing it regularly, whether you're feeling emotional or not. Find somewhere quiet to sit and in a notebook complete these sentences over and over as many times as you need to:

I feel angry with ... because

I am angry that ...

I am angry about ...

Just notice your feelings as you write and don't censor yourself. No one else will see this. Now do the same with some other sentences:

> I feel resentment that ...
>
> I feel guilty that...
>
> I'm afraid that...
>
> I'm sad that...

Again, write those sentences over and over for a few minutes, seeing what comes. Often the very act of allowing yourself to own what you feel is enough to help you start to feel better.

Whose life is it anyway? Feelings of loss

Loss is something most of us know about. At some point in our lives, someone we care about will have died and we expect to feel sadness that they have gone from our lives. When someone we know is bereaved, we treat them with compassion and gentleness.

Life as a carer is like going through a series of bereavements. First, there are the practical losses you're suffering – the hours in your day or week that are no longer available to you, the loss of income, giving up your job perhaps, losing your privacy, the end of your social life, the time to see friends.

For those of you caring for dementia sufferers, there may in addition be the 'loss' of your loved one; they are still there but no longer recognisable. And then there is the loss of your plans for your own life. Perhaps they weren't huge; you just wanted to take up gardening or learn ballroom dancing. Perhaps they were major schemes – marriage and children, a career change, backpacking round the world. Perhaps they were dreams you shared with the one who is now dependent on you – instead of a peaceful retirement you are left contemplating a lonely future looking after someone who you thought would be your soulmate.

Whether or not you're able to articulate what you want from life as clearly as that, do recognise that somewhere along the line you are having to adjust your own dreams to fit the reality of your life now as a carer. You may find yourself asking, 'Whose life is it anyway?', like James, caring for his mother, who says, 'That's what it comes down to for me. I'm living the life of a ninety-two-year-old woman.'

Treat yourself with the same compassion and gentleness you would anyone who is having to come to terms with loss on this scale. You are suffering from a major bereavement – except that unlike the bereavement that follows death, you have to face your losses anew each day.

Bereavement counsellors talk of going through stages of loss, from grief, denial, anger, guilt, depression, even despair, towards recovery. Unfortunately, because yours is a living loss, there may be no clear pathway through to 'recovery'. Rather, you feel as if you're walking in circles, experiencing the same feelings over and over.

A carers centre or online forum is a really helpful place to take those feelings and hear others tell you they understand how it feels to live with loss. But – and I shall say this a lot in this chapter – do seek professional help if you are feeling overwhelmed or stuck in a kind of feelings loop, going round and round. Many carers centres run counselling services themselves or can refer you to professionals who work with carers.

Feeling the fury

I'm not proud of this but, when I get home really tired and my son's room's in a mess, I shout at him and tell him he's no good. And of course it's not really him I'm angry with at all but

113

this whole, awful situation. The trouble is, once I've said those things the damage is done and I feel even worse.'

Sophie

This section was originally titled 'Feelings of anger'. Then I came across Marianne Talbot's wonderful account of caring for her mother, *Keeping Mum: Caring for Someone with Dementia*, and discovered at the back she'd written a whole chapter on 'Carer's Fury', a breathless, red-hot and oh-so-satisfying rant at all the 'jobsworths', lack of support, idiocy, unfairness and sheer impossibility of being a carer.

It felt good to hear another carer say out loud, 'Sometimes I am so flipping furious, so beside myself with anger, I don't know what to do with it.' (Feel free to substitute your own word for my 'flipping'.)

So, let's be honest – sometimes we *do* get angry. Our anger may be directed at ourselves, at the person we are caring for, or at the world in general. Just as when we were children we reacted angrily to things we thought were unfair, we want to stamp our foot and shout, 'This is unjust!'

If the person you're caring for is suffering, physically or emotionally, that may add to your rage. You'd take the hurt away from them if you could, and the fact that you can't, your impotence, adds fuel to the angry fires inside. And then there is the 'unacceptable' face of anger, what we sometimes feel about the person we are supposed to be taking care of. Sometimes their behaviour makes us angry. That's life – very few of us are saints.

The trouble is that in a care situation, anger doesn't feel safe. We can't express it to the person we're caring for because we know they're vulnerable. But trying to keep a lid on it really is like someone trying to contain a volcano with a plug. That's why, if your anger is sometimes directed at the person you're caring for, or may spill over into that relationship, then learning to recognise when you are boiling up, and how to deal with it, is vital – even if that means telling them you need to walk away for ten minutes to cool down.

First aid for dealing with anger

Of all the things you may be feeling, anger or fury is the most physical. That's why, in unwary hands, it can lead to playground fights, road-rage and pub punch-ups. The best ways I know to discharge the anger building up inside of you is therefore to do something physical with it – before you do anything else. As an alternative to physical anger:

- make your own punchbag from old clothes stuffed into a sack and suspended from a joist in the garage;
- buy loads of old china from a car boot sale so each time your feelings reach boiling point you can hurl a plate at the wall at the bottom of the garden;
- find a private place and rant away, loud and long;
- take a tennis racket to a cushion or pillow;
- go for a power walk, imagining the anger is pumping from your body through your hands and feet into the earth which can absorb it.

I know some carers who make a habit of taking five minutes to thump a soft pillow at the end of their bed once a week whether they feel they need to or not. Inevitably, they say after a few self-conscious punches they start to feel buried anger rising up and releasing from their bodies.

You can expect to feel self-conscious when you try any of these anger-releasing tactics, but believe me it's worth a bit of embarrassment for the rewards of feeling a sense of relief and lightness afterwards. This is usually not immediate but comes some time later when you realise you *are* feeling a fraction better for having felt, expressed and released all that emotion. That's then the time to spend a few moments assessing the situation. Ask yourself what caused your anger – a build-up of tensions or stresses, a single remark or incident? And then consider whether you need to do anything about it – tackle the cause, review the situation that's causing such difficult feelings, get more help for you? If the anger is telling you something important, those moments after you've discharged it are the time to decide if you need to take any action.

Feelings of resentment

Resentment is anger's sneaky relative – sneaky because while we sometimes allow our anger out, resentment more often festers inside, poisoning the thoughts in our head in a way that makes us feel bad about ourselves and the people around us.

If the one you're caring for doesn't seem to appreciate what you're doing for them you may well feel resentful. Or you may resent those you feel aren't helping out as much as they could – other members of your family or the professionals.

You may, in a generalised way, resent those who appear to be getting on with their lives without having the caring responsibilities that you do – colleagues, friends, neighbours, the rest of the world. Of course, you know in your head that they probably have their own trials and tribulations but still that nasty little voice hisses at you 'It's all right for them.'

Imagine you are forced to wear dark sunglasses so even on a glorious summer's day, or looking at a golden sunset, all you can see are shades of grey. Resentment is like that. It stops you seeing beauty or pleasure or even facing each new day with clear vision.

If your resentment stems from people not pulling their weight, then tell them what you feel, but do so assertively rather than resentfully.

Then park the rest – the stuff you can't do anything about because you're the one it's hurting the most.

Guilty as charged

'I feel guilty. Mum thinks I'm doing too much but my big failing is I'm not always as patient as I should be. When I'm stressed out I don't do things as well as I might. And then that makes Mum feel like she's a burden.'

Ros

And then the next moment, being the kind of person you are, you're feeling guilty for having felt anything negative at all.

Welcome to real life. Every carer I have ever spoken to feels guilty at least some of the time. Guilty that they're not doing enough for their loved ones, or enough of the right thing. Guilty that the others in their lives – partners, children, friends – are not getting enough attention. Guilty that they're not doing their work as well as they ought to because of everything else that's going on. And – in a horrible catch-22 – guilty that these feelings are sometimes being expressed in anger or resentment around their loved ones, which makes them feel even more guilty.

Guilt is one of the toughest feelings to deal with precisely because there is usually no action you can take to make the guilt go away. Unlike anger or resentment, there are no choices to be made about whether or not you say or do anything. Your guilty feelings stem from how you are judging yourself.

Which means the only one who can ever take those feelings away is also you – by choosing to stop giving yourself such a hard time, to stop judging what you do and say and recognise that you are always doing the best you can. 'Oh, but I'm not,' you tell me immediately. 'I know I could have done better in that situation. I know I wasn't doing my best.'

Actually you were. You see, if *at the time, knowing what you knew, feeling how you felt,* you could have done better, you *would* have done better or differently. Every single time we feel guilty about anything we are forgetting that simple truth and setting up some idealised version of perfection that none of us can ever attain. Let's face it, no matter how much we do for our loved ones, no matter how many somersaults we perform trying to do the right thing by everyone, it will never be enough for that inner critic.

Enough is enough. By which I mean enough guilt. Doing the best you can at any moment is enough.

All by myself

> 'Mum used to sit in the kitchen all the time and I'd sit with her where I could see the front door. It's got these wooden bars: they were like prison bars for me.'

> Janet

As a carer you may be largely housebound and feel utterly cut off and under-stimulated. Alternatively you may be the embodiment of the saying that you can feel utterly alone in a crowd; your life could hardly be busier and yet you feel completely isolated.

In either case, these feelings are likely to stem from the sense that no one understands your position. You're not getting help and everything is left to you. You are, in addition, experiencing all these difficult emotions and feel you can't share them with anyone because you think they're unacceptable.

Feelings of loneliness may also stem from loss; especially if you are caring for a partner, you may no longer have the person you used to share everything with. You don't have time to share your feelings with friends like you used to and, in any case, who'd be interested? It's not as if being a carer is exciting and gives you something to talk about!

Sometimes, our feelings of loneliness and isolation arise from believing we are unseen and undervalued. One of the most shocking findings in Carers UK's 2017 'State of Caring' report was that 73 per cent of carers feel their contribution is not valued or understood by Government or the public.

However, whether you are alone, or alone in that crowd, the remedy for loneliness or isolation *is* to reach out to others. I know that is a big ask. Admitting we're lonely can rocket us straight back to the school playground when we were the last ones to be picked for the game. It can make us feel like there's something wrong with us.

All I am asking is that you admit it to yourself, however. No one else need know. At least for now. Because you'll almost certainly find when you do allow yourself to recognise you're lonely and decide to reach out that there are plenty of people feeling exactly the way you do.

Before I give you some suggestions for how and where to reach out, a word of warning about social media. If you're housebound or severely time-limited, then social sites like Facebook can be a way of staying in touch with friends and family. But always remember it's selective. You are seeing only a snapshot of life usually – not the messy chaotic bits.

For a more realistic take on life, I recommend you join a support group run by the nearest carers centre, or find an online forum where people allow themselves to be a bit more 'real'.

Other things you could consider:

- Join a group that has nothing to do with caring – a reading group, a yoga class, or something connected to one of your hobbies or interests. I know it sounds obvious but don't forget that the important bit in deciding what to join is that the group involves some talking.

- Consider telling one or two close friends you are feeling lonely and isolated. It's perfectly possible that people stop inviting us round or out because they see our lives are impossibly busy and don't want to overload us or remind us we are missing out.

- Ask yourself which of the things we discussed is causing you to feel lonely. If you're feeling unappreciated then start appreciating yourself more. Congratulate yourself often on all you do, and reward yourself with small treats whenever you can. If your isolation is caused by the feeling you are having to do it all alone then consider how you could share more of the care. (There's a whole chapter on that coming up.)

Anxiety attack

Anxiety is not like the other feelings I've been talking about. Somehow it's an emotion we get used to living with. Of course we worry and of course we're right to be worried, we tell ourselves – who doesn't worry?

But I think anxiety has a place in this chapter on dealing with difficult emotions because long-term its effects can be just as damaging to our health and well-being. Left unchecked, anxiety can start to drive us as crazy as a tape running on endless 'repeat' in our heads. It can rob us of sleep when it becomes our mind crashing into gear at 2 a.m. Or stop us enjoying the good things of life, because how can we when there is so much to worry about?

Anxiety is exhausting and debilitating. It is also, quite often, pointless, which is why I want to share one of the best ways I know of handling your worries if you become aware that you are driving yourself mad with anxiety.

No worries

Keep an exercise book or journal nearby and when you catch your mind running on a soundtrack of worry and anxiety complete the following exercise:

Today's date ..../......../..........

These are my worries: ....

....

....

....

....

Can I do something about them?

Yes – here is my plan:

....

....

....

....

....

No? Then I give myself permission to stop thinking about them.

Should I get help?

If you fear your feelings are in danger of running out of control, if they seem unmanageable or out of proportion to what's going on, if you think there is a chance of you lashing out at someone else, you have reached a point where you need to get support. In the same way that animals instinctively react to a looming storm by seeking shelter, long before there is any obvious sign of the danger to come, our feelings are our early warning systems. If this is true for you, turn to Chapters 14 and 15 on sharing care and getting support for you for advice on where to get help right now.

On the other hand, you may find allowing yourself to acknowledge and accept your feelings – and forgiving yourself for having them – takes away some of their power to damage you. The energy that you've been spending keeping the lid on them is now available for you to direct into more positive areas of your life.

Copy or cut out the Carer's Creed below and stick it beside your bed so you can look at it every morning before the day starts and every night when the day is done.

Carer's Creed

- Whatever you feel able to do is enough
- Things don't have to be perfect – drop your standards
- Treat yourself with the same gentleness and understanding that you would another carer
- Negative feelings don't make you a bad person; they mean you're in a bad situation
- You're not a saint – don't let other people's expectations get in the way of you doing the best you can
- Work out what you can and can't change, and stop worrying about everything in the 'can't' column

---

CHAPTER 13
Survival

'My mental health was very badly affected by the need to make decisions for someone who was incapacitated by dementia and was very verbally vicious. At times, I felt so angry and upset by the injustice of it.'

Ingrid

We've looked at dealing with some of the difficult emotions caring may bring up. But what if it's worse than that? What if it's you, the carer, who is in crisis?

I'm very wary of scaring you, dear reader. After all, there are many carers for whom their role is often a positive experience, and even when it isn't they somehow manage to keep calm and carry on. The vast majority of carers don't reach breaking point or experience the kind of burnout which stopped my sister and me in our tracks. But I'd be lying if I hid from you that a fair number of carers I've interviewed did experience their own crises.

Depression, despair, co-dependency, burnout, breakdown – I truly hope that they never happen to you. If they do – and there is nothing wrong with that; you haven't failed – perhaps this chapter will help.

Understanding depression and despair

Feeling emotional is understandable. Experiencing some of the emotions we've talked about fairly regularly is pretty normal for carers. What you need to watch out for are feelings of hopelessness and despair which are warning signs that you may be suffering from depression.

Depression is a medical condition. It may have been triggered by some of the factors we've discussed, by physical and emotional overload as a result of being a carer. But it's medical help you need first to prevent your condition getting worse and even affecting your ability to go on caring.

Among the signs that you may be suffering from depression are:

- You feel sad, lonely and anxious all the time
- You're not sure what gets you up in the morning
- You feel angry with everyone
- No matter what you do, you feel it's not enough
- The slightest demand sends you screaming into the corner
- You can't remember when you last laughed
- You can't seem to make a decision about anything
- Sometimes you think it would be easier to die
- You have suicidal thoughts.

Although seeking support with your caring role and for yourself will help in time, one of the insidious symptoms of depression is its power to rob you of the energy, will and confidence to take such action. So if you recognise you're at risk or already suffering from depression, the first step is always to see your doctor.

Alongside that get in touch with your local carers centre who will certainly be able to put you in touch with a range of support services, including professional counselling. Or contact one of the mental-health support groups listed in the resource section at the back of the book – they have so much experience of handling depression and coming out the other side.

How to recognise stress

Scientists say a little stress is good for us, but they're not talking about the sort of things that are probably stressing you. What you need to know is that stress that runs on day after day, year after year, can be very dangerous to your health. It raises blood pressure, reduces your immunity to germs and can ultimately lead to burnout (what used to be known as 'a nervous breakdown').

Stress expresses itself in a huge number of different ways. Take a look at the list below. If you tick more than three or four of these symptoms you've probably reached the stage of needing to review your caring role, make some changes, seek support or get medical help before you get sick.

- You wake in the night worrying and find it impossible to switch off
- You have real trouble getting to sleep in the first place
- You're drinking more alcohol, smoking more cigarettes or eating more of the wrong foods than is good for you
- You get tearful at what seem to be small things
- People and situations irritate you far more than they used to
- Your mood sometimes swings wildly but your highs and lows are not necessarily related to what's going on
- You suffer from headaches, high blood pressure, sickness, loss of appetite, muscular twitches, rashes
- You feel exhausted all the time
- You feel stretched to breaking point
- You've stopped enjoying things that used to give you pleasure
- You catch every virus that is going around.

Setting boundaries

'If Mum's having a bad day, then so am I. I might have left her and be back in my own front room but she's there in the back of my mind the whole time and I can't relax and let it go.'

Rose

One of the definitions of co-dependency is when your quality of life is dependent on the quality of life of another. As Melody Beattie explains in her book *Codependent No More: How to Stop Controlling Others and Start Caring for Yourself,* we are co-dependent when we have lost sight of our own lives: 'When I asked them what they were feeling, they told me what the other person was feeling. When I asked what they did, they told me what the other person had done.'

Of course, there are degrees of this. We all want our loved ones to be OK. Yet getting so drawn in that our own happiness and well-being are entirely hostage to that of someone else is deeply damaging to our physical and mental health – even to our ability to continue as carers.

When do we need to do less caring and practise more self-care? How do we set boundaries to ensure we survive, too?

If you are struggling to think of your life as in any way separate from your role as a carer it may be time to set some limits for yourself. Once again, I'm going to ask you to write down your answers to these questions. When we answer them in our heads it's much easier to forget them, and forget to do them. You matter. Make this time to reconnect with your own life.

1. **Refocus on your own happiness** – what are the things that made you happy in the past? What occupations absorb you so much that you forget about everything else? Answer these questions in at least five ways. Now choose at least two or three things that you are willing to commit to doing regularly.

2. **Be honest about where your responsibilities for your loved one begin and end** – now write down what you are responsible for. Their safety, finances, personal care, whatever your caring role entails. Now write down what you can't be responsible for – their happiness, how long they live, how they behave, etc. Trust me on this: none of us has the power to make another happy or healthy or grateful, etc. We go crazy when we try to take that on, too. Writing this down in black and white may help you actually see it is true.

3. **Weigh up the balance of care** – thinking about a typical day or week or month in your life, how much time do you spend caring for your loved one (and others, too) and how much for yourself? Answer honestly. Now I want you to write down the precise ways in which you practise self-care. If, as I suspect, the scales are heavily tipped in favour of caring for others, ask yourself how long you expect a battery to last if it is rarely charged? List some self-care strategies and commit to them, even if it means you're a little less available for others.

4. **Learn acceptance** – one of my favourite writers, Byron Katie, says that most of our pain comes from wanting things to be different from the way they are. Arguing with reality in other words. We tell ourselves things shouldn't be this way, people shouldn't get ill, there should be more help available, and all the time those thoughts are sending us a little more crazy because very often we can't actually do anything to change the way things are. Remember the words of the Serenity Prayer: 'Grant me the serenity to accept the things I cannot change, the courage to change what I can, and the wisdom to know the difference.' Remind yourself often that acceptance is the pathway to peace.

Changing your thinking

Practising acceptance means changing how you think about the things that are going on in your life. And it's worth pointing out that changing your thinking is a useful tactic at every stage as a carer.

Over the years of caring for Mum, so much of my stress came from the thought that I never had time. From the moment I walked through the door, there was so much that needed doing – cooking, tidying up, tackling the latest bills – and on top of that Mum wanted an outing. Aargh!

It took me a long time to realise that even thinking the thought that there wasn't enough time simply added to my stress. So I chose to replace that stress thought with something that helped me feel a little better – 'Everything that matters gets done'. Somehow that helped me slow down a bit and, miraculously, when I stopped trying to rush myself and rush Mum things did get done, just as they always had. Only with less strain.

The same practice has helped me with my thoughts about being a carer. Sometimes, I would catch myself inwardly railing at the injustice of finding myself in this position, not once but twice, and the unfairness of Mum getting sick just as my oldest child was leaving home and I was looking forward to 'me time'. I'd catch my own soundtrack, chuntering unhappily on about the inadequacy of the care Mum was getting, or the horror of having to clean up another accident.

Guess what? The more I thought those things the worse *I* felt.

Don't get me wrong; I'm not saying any of those challenges we face as carers are OK. Only that when our thoughts run riot on all that is wrong, it's us who suffer the most.

You won't always manage it, but every time you can turn one of those stress thoughts around and remind yourself of one small positive about your caring role, you'll be helping yourself to feel a fraction better.

May I start you off with a few kinder thoughts that are 100 per cent true:

- You are doing an amazing job
- You are making a difference
- Every day you are a carer you are making the world a fractionally kinder and more loving place
- We are grateful to you
- Thank you.

CHAPTER 14

Hundreds of Ways to Get Help

'Caregiving takes a village.'

Susanne White, founder of www.caregiverwarrior.com,
from her e-book *The Caregiver's Little Guide to Survival:
7 Fail-Safe Tips for Caregivers*

You heard what Susanne said – just like bringing up a child, caring for someone takes a whole village.

Well, that's great, you think, so where is this village? Where are the people who are supposed to be helping me? How is it that I seem to be stuck out here on my own?

Believe me, I sympathise. But I'm also going to suggest that if the village won't come to you, you need to find the energy and willpower to go out and find it.

Why? Here's the rest of the quote from Susanne: 'Trying to do all of it alone is overwhelming and exhausting, and we can begin to feel crazy and emotionally bankrupt. This is a breeding ground for bad decisions, isolation and loneliness. It's crazy-making.'

In this chapter, I'm going to make some suggestions about who and what's available in that village and how you can get them involved in sharing the caring – for the sake of your loved one, but for your sake above all.

Paid carers and care agencies

Preparing meals, cleaning, shopping, gardening, keeping your loved one clean, getting them up, getting them dressed, answering their call during the night – these are just some of the daily tasks you could consider sharing with paid carers. There is now a huge number of agencies set up to enable people who need support to stay in their homes for as long as they possibly can.

But how do you find a good agency? If you can, start by consulting other carers. Ask on one of the forums if anyone can recommend an agency in your area. Speak to carers at your carers centre. Talk to every friend and neighbour who lives in your area – someone somewhere will know of someone who is using a care agency.

Have a look at their websites and try and get a sense for what they prioritise. But remember – words can come cheap. And even within each agency there are likely to be good and less good carers. After all, they're as individual as we are.

When 'interviewing' an agency, these are a few of the questions you might want to ask:

- Will my loved one see the same carers most of the time? What happens if a carer is sick or there is an emergency? A good agency will try to minimise the number of different carers coming into your loved one's home.
- How do you select your carers, how long do they stay and how do you monitor the work and care your staff give? Good staff will be attracted to good agencies that treat them well and maintain standards. High turnover of staff is a sure sign that all is not well.

- What formal qualifications do you require your staff to have and what training do you provide for them? For instance, are they supported to learn about treating people with dignity and respect, about first aid, healthy eating, manual handling and so on? Good agencies will invest in their staff.
- How will you communicate with me about my loved one's care? Even if they take over many of the care tasks, you remain a partner in your loved one's care. A good agency recognises this and will check in with you regularly.
- Finally, check the agency is registered with the Care Quality Commission in England, the Regulation and Quality Improvement in Northern Ireland, the Care Inspectorate (in Scotland) or Care and Social Services Inspectorate Wales, and with the United Kingdom Homecare Association, which requires its members to sign up to a code of practice to ensure high standards.

How will we pay for this care?

If you haven't already contacted the local council and requested a care assessment, then now's the time. The assessment will help you identify which tasks in the care plan *could* be done by someone else and what, if anything, the council is obliged to pay towards the cost of that help.

If your loved one has enough financial assets not to qualify for any help in paying for care services, the council can still help you by managing the contract with the agency on your behalf, which saves you some of the bureaucracy. Besides which, you're getting yourselves on their radar. Your loved one's care, and how it's paid for, should be reviewed annually in any case, but if funds start to run low it will be quicker and easier to bring them in for a review to trigger more financial support.

Just remember, as you gaze at an invoice for seemingly crazy amounts of money for what you have been doing for 'free' – it's never been for free. There is a cost to you in terms of all of the challenges we've been talking about in this book.

Remember, too, if they qualify for attendance allowance, that it's there to help with these additional expenses. It's also true that if your loved one does have assets, they've been accumulated at least in part for 'a rainy day'. Guess what – this is it. This is the unforeseen thing they put money aside for. What better way to use it than on helping you to help them and yourself?

How do I know whether it's working?

Do introduce a paid carer slowly if you can, perhaps when you are going to be away for a day or two. And once you've done so, take the time to ask your loved one how it is working and listen to them. Ask them to describe how they are cared for – what happens during a care visit, how are they treated and spoken to, and how do they feel.

Your loved one's mood and – unless they have advanced dementia – what they say about the carers will be one of your best indicators of how well it is working. If your loved one is resistant to the idea of anyone caring for them other than you, then you may not hear an accurate story, only the truth as they see it. But look out for any change in their behaviour or nature. If you spot any unexplained changes, then you need to find out what is going on.

It's always a good idea, too, to drop in unexpectedly just to see if people are turning up on time and how they are handling things. At the same time, remember that, just like you, paid carers usually have too much to do and too little time to do it. They have good days and bad days, too. Most are hugely dedicated to work which pays poorly and involves unsocial hours. Get to know them and let them get to know you. That will build trust on all sides, and ensure that when something is amiss your gut alerts you so you can take action.

Day centres and lunch clubs

'I thought Dad would be upset when the health visitor said she'd try and get him a few days at the hospice, but he used to look forward to those days so much. They'd offer him a bath if he wanted, which was wonderful because he could only manage a shower at home. And before they served lunch – which was all properly set out with tablecloths and flowers on the table – they always offered him a glass of sherry. He said it was like going to dinner in a hotel.'

Brian

Day centres can be wonderful places, geared to providing interest, activity and support for people of varying ages and with a range of conditions. The best day centres also bring in local schools and colleges, entertainers and musicians to broaden the programme and ensure the right sort of variety. Some are run by the social services or education departments of your local council, some by charities such as Age UK, and some as adjuncts to private care homes.

If your loved one has cancer or a life-limiting illness they may qualify to attend a day centre at a local hospice. Like other centres, these are activity-based, offering everything from occupational therapy, arts and crafts to massage and hairdressing. Many day centres also offer attended transport to and from their base.

The best way of accessing these facilities is through that care plan again, or via a referral from social services or the doctor. Or you could contact the nearest branch of Age UK or your nearest carers centre to find out who's running what day services in your area. If a day centre doesn't suit, there are almost certain to be lunch clubs, either run by Age UK, or through council sheltered housing schemes, that welcome all-comers.

Even one day a week (or the few hours of a lunch club) can have a positive effect on you both – for them, attending regularly brings a new circle of faces into their life; for you, a bit of time to call (mostly) your own.

Holidays and respite

I've put these together because sometimes they can be the same thing. A holiday for them – respite for you. At other times, respite might be provided within a local care or nursing home, where your loved one will stay as a temporary resident so you can have a break from caring.

So let's start with holidays. A number of wonderful charities offer holiday packages, either for the person you care for by themselves, or for you to go together.

If you, the person you care for, or both of you, badly need a break, together or from each other, turn to the resources section at the back of this book for some suggestions on where to look. Some places will require you to accompany the person you care for, but provide plenty of support to ensure you get a bit of a break, too. Others will act as stand-in carers, with trained staff taking over your caring role for a week or two.

A good source of information may be any charity set up to support people with the specific condition your loved one has. Mencap, for instance, organises holidays for unaccompanied children and adults and publishes a holiday accommodation guide to places where people with a learning disability are welcome.

If you do arrange a holiday for the person you're caring for, you may be tempted simply to curl up and stay at home while they're away.

That's fine, unless you discover you're so used to being frantically busy you end up using the time to catch up on other jobs. Don't! If there's one certainty in life, it is that no matter how much you do, the jobs are never complete. It will do you so much more good to have a complete rest. If you must be busy, find some sort of relaxing activity instead – get out, visit a local museum or gallery, arrange to have coffee with friends.

And do consider taking a holiday yourself. Don't you deserve to have someone preparing and clearing up *your* meals, not even having to make your own bed if you don't want to?

If you know you need some kind of break from caring, then start by talking to your social or case worker – the people who did your assessment. They may have agreed a certain number of weeks' respite each year to support you in your caring role – and if they haven't, now may be the time to get it written into an updated carer's assessment. They will have an arrangement with a number of local residential care or nursing homes where your loved one could become a temporary resident for a week or two. It will usually be down to the council to organise it, even if – depending on their age and assets – your loved one has to pay for it.

And with an eye on the possible long-term, it's a chance for you to learn a little more about how some of the local residential homes operate and how good they are at what they do. There's more on residential care in Chapter 17.

I'd be lying if I said getting respite is easy. It's really not. Even when it is written into the plan. If it's the council you are struggling to convince then you are going to have to take a deep breath and tell it like it is. You may have practical reasons for wanting time out from caring – wanting to take your children on holiday, or meet some other important commitment in your life. The Carer's Act says you are entitled to support in getting on with the parts of your life that are important.

If you are simply at the end of your tether then say so; tell the social worker or doctor that without a break you're in danger of getting ill which will mean they'll have to take over the entire caring role.

Another respite route to consider, if the person you care for objects to going away, may be to bring in a live-in carer on a temporary basis and go away yourself. In order to do this, there must be a spare bedroom in the house where the live-in carer can stay.

Family and friends

Of course there is another group that could provide respite – relatives and friends. Before you dismiss the idea – because, after all, if your relatives were interested they'd have shown up long before now – re-read the chapter on relationships. Perhaps your family wouldn't be comfortable splitting up the work on a daily basis, but they would be willing to bring your loved one into their own homes for a few days so you have a break. Or, if that's impractical for any reason, they might consider coming to stay in your loved one's home for a short time and take over your care duties.

As for friends, many of those who say earnestly, 'Tell me if there is anything I can do to help,' *actually mean it.* Knowing what's involved in being a carer, you may feel reluctant to involve friends, but remind yourself you're not asking them to do what you do. You're only asking them to give you a few hours' break.

And it's surprising how small amounts of help add up. If you're used to only getting one hour to yourself a day (and that will seem generous to some carers), then an extra two or three hours' help a week is a significant improvement. Ask them if they'd be willing to sit with your loved one for two hours once a week, keeping them company, ensuring they're safe and carrying out just a few of the basic tasks, such as preparing a meal.

What if my loved one objects?

Sometimes, the biggest obstacle to sharing the caring is that your loved one – who, after all, is the one who may have to pay – objects. That's OK if you really are superhuman and plan never to get ill, tired, fretful, or in any way unable to be a carer temporarily.

But you're not. And what will happen if you don't get help is that you'll become ill and they'll have to put up with other carers whether they like it or not.

Take a deep breath and be clear and honest with them that if you don't get more help and the occasional break you're worried you won't be able to go on caring. It may not be ideal – but they'll survive and be looked after. What's more, in a relationship that is probably one-sided, agreeing to something that will help you is one way in which they can give *you* some care back.

Sometimes, it's change people are scared of and, once they get used to a professional carer coming in, or to spending a week once or twice a year in respite care, they may welcome the break, and the new faces, as much as you do.

After all, you may be the most fascinating person in the world but if you're the only one your loved one gets to see and talk to every day, that fascination may become a little jaded.

Other paid help

'It became obvious Mum wasn't managing to look after the house so, after we went in and did a cleaning blitz, we persuaded her she needed a home help, which she still has. The next thing was food. I was spending two or three hours there every evening cooking dinner. Now we've found someone to come in to do dinner four times a week which means I

get home earlier those evenings. It's paid for out of Mum's attendance allowance.'

Rob

Not every job you are currently doing needs a paid carer to do it in place of you. It really is worth keeping an audit for a week of all the things you are currently doing for your loved one, then asking yourself if there are jobs others could be brought in to take on, such as help around the house. It could cover anything or everything from cleaning, tidying, washing, ironing, shopping to cooking and washing up.

If your loved one has the resources to pay for it then think about how much time and energy that would free up for you to focus on the bits of your caring role that really matter to you. And if they can't, and they're receiving attendance allowance, those are precisely the things it's intended for.

There are some truly wonderful home helps out there who, in time, may become a really significant and valued member of your small 'care team' – as well as a friend to your loved one.

CHAPTER 15

Getting Support for You

'I often say that those of us who commit to caregiving are in it for the long haul. We don't give in and we don't give up. We are hardwired to take this responsibility very seriously and will do everything we can to ensure that our loved ones are comfortable and safe. We must be as committed to our own well-being and health as we are to the well-being of our loved ones. Only then will we be able to have moments when we enjoy the powerful and intense caregiving journey.'

Susanne White, founder of www.caregiverwarrior.com, from her e-book *The Caregiver's Little Guide to Survival: 7 Fail-Safe Tips for Caregivers*

For years, I resisted the idea of paying a cleaner to give my home even a basic once-over each week. I should be able to fit it in somehow, I thought, and then another week would go by and, as I rushed around trying to be a working single parent and carer, I'd feel I was failing badly because my children and I were going home to a dirty house.

It was the same with caring for myself. If I wasn't busy being a carer for my uncle, then I needed to put extra effort into being a mother to two under tens and to my job. It wasn't that people didn't offer to help. They did. But mostly I didn't believe they meant it. Or I didn't want to put *them* out.

The terms 'superwoman' and 'superman' are not compliments but burdens – trying to live up to them is simply another load on our backs. The sooner we allow ourselves to accept that self-care has to be at least as much a priority as caring for our loved one, the better it will be for both our physical and emotional health.

You see, with just about everything you do in life, from sewing to learning Swahili, the more you practise, the better you get. Except caring. You may well get better at it in the sense of being more able to juggle all the competing demands or change a bandage more quickly. But far from getting easier, most carers find it gets harder with each passing day.

The reason is not hard to fathom. We are like cars in the fast lane, taking on more, operating on adrenalin. But if you sit too long in the fast lane, you start to get tired and the fuel begins to run out. That's why they invented service areas, to give us a chance to rest, refuel and service our vehicles. There are service areas for carers, too, but unlike those you'll find on the motorway they're not always easy to spot. Nor will you see signposts telling you 'Tiredness kills – take a break'.

Finding and asking for help

In the last chapter, we looked at some of your choices for sharing the caring. This section is about getting help for *you* from a range of informal sources, whether you need a chat, the company of people who understand, tips and advice, or a more sustained programme of counselling or emotional support.

Before we look at useful sources of support, try the quiz below to help you recognise how easy – or not – you find it is to ask for help. Be sure to answer the questions honestly – this is for your benefit, no one else's.

How Easy Do You Find It to Ask for Help?

For each question, honestly mark the response that you are most likely to give:

1. **You're meeting a friend outside the post office in a town you've not visited before and you're already ten minutes late. Do you:**
   a) ring his mobile, apologise for being late and ask him for directions;
   b) head for the town centre and, when you haven't found the post office after a few minutes, stop someone to ask;
   c) weave your way around the town centre until you spot the sign, even though you're now twenty minutes overdue.

2. **At the supermarket, when the cashier asks if you need any help packing, do you:**
   a) say, 'Yes please'– four hands are obviously better than two;
   b) decline, unless there's already someone standing there – you wouldn't want to upset them;
   c) always say, 'No' – no one else packs the way you like it done.

3. **You bump into a neighbour who says they haven't seen you for a while and asks how you are. Do you:**
   a) admit that you've been tied up caring for a loved one and that although you want to do it you are finding it a struggle;
   b) agree you've not been home much lately then ask them how they are;
   c) smile and say, 'I'm fine, thank you.'

4. **Your busiest friend is organising a surprise birthday party for her husband but when she phones to invite you and hears about your life she says, 'Let me know if there's anything I can do to help . . .' Do you:**

   a) thank her and suggest that after the party you'll call her to discuss how she can help;

   b) say, 'Oh, you've got far too much on your plate,' but decide if she disagrees or offers again you might find a job for her to do;

   c) change the subject back to the party – offering to help is just something people do to be polite; they don't really mean it.

5. **A social worker comes to see you and suggests you need a break. She says she'll arrange respite care for your loved one but, after three weeks, you've not heard anything. Do you:**

   a) phone her on her direct line to ask whether she has managed to set something up;

   b) assume that no news is bad news – if she'd been able to do something, you would have heard by now;

   c) shrug – it's what you expected. They never seem able to deliver what they say they will.

Have a look at your answers and if you got:

Mostly (a)s: Well done. Even if you'd rather manage alone, you've learned how to ask for help and recognise your own limitations. The chances are you've already made efforts to get yourself some support in your caring role. But take a look at the suggestions below to see if there's any more help you could access.

Mostly (b)s: You seem to recognise that you need help but your sensitivity to everyone else's feelings is preventing you from being direct about your needs. Take a look back at the section on assertiveness (Chapter 4) and, remember, carers need care, too. Being able to ask for help is a sign of strength, not weakness.

Mostly (c)s: Poor you. It sounds as if any attempts you've made to get help have ended in disappointment and you'd rather not ask at all than have to deal with being let down again. It will take a lot of courage to change your attitude and look for help. You could start gently by accepting any offers that come your way, and by reminding yourself the best-tuned engine will judder to a halt when it runs out of fuel.

If your answers were mainly (b)s and (c)s ask yourself what the barriers are that stop you from asking for help and getting support for you personally. Is it embarrassment at being seen as needy, fear of being told no or let down, is it habit (you've always managed somehow), funds (you don't have money to spend on yourself), or pig-headedness? It may be a combination of those things, which is all fine and good – except that you're the one paying the penalty for going it alone.

However you answered, it may help to consider the following:

- It takes far more courage to ask for help than to go on until you drop. We know you're strong. Dare you be strong enough to seek and ask for support?
- A useful way of expressing your need for help is to agree with whoever you're asking that you have their permission to ask on

the understanding they have your permission to say no. That will help you both be honest.

- Learn to distinguish do-ers from say-ers. As the saying goes, if you want something done, ask a busy person.
- Don't underestimate the value of small acts of helping. Someone watering the garden once a week frees up fifteen minutes you could spend on a phone call to a friend or having an afternoon nap.
- It's not personal – if someone turns you down or agrees to help and then doesn't deliver it's down to them, nothing to do with you. Tell yourself it's not intended to hurt you, remember not to ask them again, and let it go.
- Don't feel guilty. Think for a moment about how you feel when you're able to help someone, even if it's only someone stopping you in the street and asking for directions. Most of us get a gentle glow from knowing we're being helpful. Don't deprive others of that!

Join a carers centre or support group

'We get ideas from each other. This chap has a mentally ill daughter who's lying in bed all the time and I said so was my son, so I moved his bed into another room, away from the telly and computer. A week later he said that worked – she has to get up now.'

Jenny

Actions don't always speak louder than words. Practical help is wonderful, but so too is sitting down with someone and knowing that every word you say will be not just understood but accepted in the right spirit. To the rest of the world you may hesitate to admit how truly bad it sometimes gets. But among other carers, and those who support them, you know everything you say is safe.

To find out if there is a carers centre in your area, speak to the adult social care team, call the local library, ask at your doctor's surgery, or contact one of the national carers organisations listed in the resources section. If that doesn't yield anything, you could think about starting up your own support group! Yes, I know you're already impossibly busy, but you'll still be just as busy whether you make time for a group or not. That's how it works with carers. And think about what you'll get from a support group:

- **empathy** – the comfort of being with people who know what you're going through even if you don't feel like talking about it.
- **honesty** – to be yourself and share your experience with no one sitting in judgement.
- **advice** – if you want it from those who have been there, done that, and got a wardrobe full of T-shirts.
- **humour** – it's possible that only with other carers will you find relief in laughing about the impossible, the awful and the ridiculous.
- **hope** – listening to other people's problems can take some of the sting out of yours, and offer solutions to problems you thought had none.

Apart from contact with other carers, centres offer access to a whole range of other support services; for instance, one group has arranged for former carers to ring current carers every morning, just to make sure that every single day they have someone they can offload to if they wish – someone caring about *them*.

My nearest centre offers everything from massage and meditation, through outings and practical problem-solving, to education and training, as Maurice discovered: 'The carers group paid for me to do a creative writing course with the National Extension College and loaned a computer so I could write poetry and short stories. When you first go, you think they're all going to be down and miserable but they're not. Most of the people I've met have a lot of energy and don't feel sorry for themselves at all.'

Get connected

These days not all networks are physical. The advent of the Internet has made possible the creation of a myriad of new networks reflecting people's needs and interests – and naturally that includes carers. If your caring responsibilities mean you are often housebound do consider what help you could get online. All of the major carers organisations have websites where you'll not only find loads of useful information but also other carers sharing tips and tribulations and offering support to each other. And being the Internet, of course, you are not limited to this country. You can drop in on support groups anywhere around the globe if you fancy expanding your horizons.

For many carers, 'online' means 'lifeline'. If you think it would make a difference to you, but buying and running a decent mobile phone, tablet or computer is beyond you financially, it's well worth looking at whether you could get a grant from a charity, or even from social services, to help you get connected. If all else fails, your local library may be under threat but it will have computers you can use, usually free of charge.

One more thing you will find online is a number of stroppy carers – and that's good news. These are folk who sometimes feel the same anger, frustration and despair as the rest of us but have found that channelling those emotions into campaigning for a better deal for carers is an excellent outlet for their strong feelings.

If there are times when you find yourself spitting with fury about some professional's inability to return a phone call, about the abysmal level of funding with which social services is expected to support carers, or about the pittance carer's allowance represents, try venting your spleen in an email to your MP, to the PM, or to the Government department where these decisions are made. It can be every bit as therapeutic as beating your pillow to death – with one difference. In the privacy of your own home, no one can hear you scream. Online, or in the post, as part of a national campaign, your cry for help may be echoed a thousand times over until it can't *not* be heard.

Seek counselling

'My mum, nan and grandad, who I'd been caring for, died within five weeks of each other and I had panic attacks. I was at A&E every week thinking I was having a heart attack. The doctor suggested a counsellor and, to start with, I bit her head off because she was trying to tell me I was suffering from stress! Of course, before long I knew she was right ... she's really helped me see what was wrong.'

Teresa

There are many ways to access counselling. Your doctor may recommend it if your feelings are really starting to get on top of you or you're suffering stress overload. Some carers centres can put you in touch with a counsellor, or offer counselling sessions themselves. Or you can locate services privately in your area.

Alternatively, contact the British Association for Counselling who'll be able to give you the names of accredited professionals near your home. And don't be put off if you live in the back of beyond. Increasingly, some counsellors now offer sessions over the phone or online using services such as Skype.

Deciding to have a few counselling sessions may feel like a big step for a coper, but it's really no different from asking a doctor for help with a medical problem you can't resolve by yourself. The important thing to remember is to be absolutely clear with yourself and the counsellor why you are there. This is almost certainly not the time to be digging deep into the past, looking back at all the troubling things which are now part of your DNA. What you need from these sessions is an emotional workout that will help you survive – and even thrive – as a carer.

Many counselling services are run by charities who are happy to work for a heavily reduced rate with people on low incomes. Usually, you'll be asked to agree with your counsellor what you can afford. The service may even be free of charge if you're referred by a doctor or by another professional.

And don't forget the Samaritans, whose phone line operates twenty-four hours a day, seven days a week. Their trained volunteers are there to listen to anyone in distress or in need of emotional support.

Phone the family, phone a friend

There are any number of reasons why you may feel you're not getting any support from other relatives or friends of yours, or of the person you're caring for.

The least charitable explanation is that they're just darn lazy and quite happy for you to carry the load, thank you very much. But, let's be honest, although we all know such sloths, most people are decent – just busy and stressed and trying to juggle their commitments the same as you are.

The answer is to involve a lot of people in doing little things – which adds up to a decent amount of help for you. For instance, if your relatives always phone you for news of the person you're caring for, couldn't you agree to make just one call to one relative and then they can pass the news on to everyone else?

Take a look at some of the suggestions below for ways in which others might help, and add your own items or start your own list. By producing it you are making it safe for people to offer a hand, giving them the chance to choose to support you in a way that fits in with their lives.

You can also show the list, or suggest items from it, to those friends who offer to help. Remember, most people are genuine and, if the boot was on the other foot and you could see one of your friends going under, wouldn't you be first in the queue with a homemade casserole or a handkerchief?

Help List

- Spare a few hours once a week or once a month to sit with my loved one so I can get out
- Take them for a drive from time to time
- Come and read to them from a book or the newspaper on a regular basis
- Bring cards or a board game to play with them
- Bring books and music from the library and then change them regularly
- Bring a pet to visit
- Do my shopping
- Clean my car
- Make an extra portion of dinner to put in the freezer for me
- Help with my gardening
- Help with my housework
- Take my children for an outing
- Invite me for a quick coffee
- Arrange a night out for me
- Pay for me to have a back and neck massage
- Keep me company one day when I'm being a carer

Extreme self-care

I've used this term deliberately because I want to drive home how little self-care you are most likely managing on. It was invented by Cheryl Richardson, whose books *Stand Up for Your Life* and *Take Time for Your Life* I heartily recommend. They are packed with good advice on honouring your own needs, learning what you need to say 'No' to and how to do that, and being true to yourself.

In the meantime, here are a few questions to help you identify the ways in which you need to care for yourself better:

- What does my body need to feel nurtured, strong and healthy? For example, it might be drinking lots of water, making time for exercise, choosing healthier foods, getting to bed earlier.
- Who can I turn to for support? Who's in my support network? What do I need from them? How can I make time to share my feelings with them?
- Who and what do I need to avoid? Who increases my anxiety level or drains my energy? What are the situations that bring me down? What do I need to let go of?
- What unhelpful coping strategies do I need to avoid? For instance, drinking too much, eating too much sugar or working too late into the night.
- If a doctor said my life depended on me treating myself better, what would I change? What would I start doing? What would I stop doing? Guess what, your life *does* depend on it.

Here are some responses from carers in answer to the question 'How do you support yourself?':

- 'I recently began making jewellery and writing poetry. I find both therapeutic.'
- 'I go to bed at seven every night and get as much sleep as I can.'
- 'Mandatory *me* time – mainly for massages.'

- 'Coffee with friends and rare weekends away.'
- 'I go to church.'
- 'Wine, reading, walking the dogs.'
- 'Yoga, exercise and meditation.'
- 'I try to keep physically healthy and strong.'
- 'My family are very supportive so I talk to them about my concerns.'
- 'Alternative therapies, vitamins and forgiveness!'
- 'I arrange to have a walking weekend with my best friend every other month. It saves my sanity.'
- 'I start every day journalling, just to see what's on my mind and get it out of my system.'

CHAPTER 16

Review, Review, Review

'Looking back, Mum should have gone into a home about six months ago ... But I was arrogant enough to believe that no one could look after her as well as I could, frightened by our dreadful experience of respite and, frankly, I was too exhausted to be able to see straight.'

Marianne Talbot in *Keeping Mum: Caring for Someone with Dementia*

In almost ten years now of caring for Mum, I can tell you that the only thing we've ever been able to be sure of is that things change. Our loved one changes, their condition changes, we change, and all around us life changes, too.

Every time we have got into a rhythm, known where we are with the caring for a few weeks or months, something happens to throw all the cards back up in the air. The same will be true for you, which is why it's so important to keep all your decisions, routines, expectations and choices under review.

Stop, look, listen to see what's changed

When we're under pressure, we're also often on 'automatic'. That makes it much harder to notice immediately if arrangements or choices that once worked are no longer working so well. There's also the comfort of what's become familiar. Knowing where we are as carers makes it a little easier to plan the rest of our lives – rather than having to start the juggling all over again.

I've lost count of the number of times my sister and I have had to adjust our working and personal routines to fit with a change in Mum's condition and capabilities, and with our own ability to cope. Sometimes it's been thrust on us – such as when Mum slipped and fractured a femur and suddenly the walking frame had to be replaced with a wheelchair and all that entails. At other times, it's crept up on us – as when we realised the cost of doing all the care visits ourselves had become so overwhelming that my sister was close to breaking point. We were long past the point of needing to bring in paid carers to take some of the load from us.

I hope you do better than us at remembering to keep every aspect of your life as a carer under review. For instance:

- The decisions you made for your loved one's care may have been rushed by circumstances. In the light of experience and without that urgency, do they still look like the right decisions?
- Life moves on. Perhaps the person you're caring for needs more help or less help than they did. Are the arrangements you made still best for them and you?
- And what about all the other parts of your life: family, friends, dependants, work? Has anything changed there which you now need to take into account?
- Perhaps when you started caring you didn't know there were alternatives or that it might be possible to get more help. Are there changes that would benefit one or both of you?

Let me tell you about Bernadette, who cared for her father for more than a decade while her three sisters got on with having families, jobs and social lives. It wasn't that they loved their father less; simply that one by one they left home to get married until Bernadette was the only one still living with their father.

The unthinkable happened when Bernadette arranged for her sisters to cover for her for a fortnight while she took her first solo holiday in years. A few days into her break she met an American living in France. By the time the fortnight was up, Bernadette had fallen in love and decided she was moving to France to get married, and someone else would have to look after her father.

The moral of this story is that no matter how tied you feel to the current care arrangements, life can still catch you out. For us as carers, there are rarely simple or easy choices — only the choice we make at the time. For ten years, Bernadette's choice was to be a carer until the day came when her choice was to go on caring about her father's well-being but put her own happiness first.

If you suddenly announced you couldn't go on, someone, somewhere, most probably within the professional health and social services, would have to pick up the pieces.

Recognising when something needs to change

The questions that follow are intended to guide your thoughts and give you a chance to reflect. They do cover some areas that you may find difficult, or may make you feel emotional. If so, try and get help working through the list, either from a trusted friend, or from a professional such as a counsellor.

Remember, you are doing this review for you and your loved one, but you don't need to share it with them. You need to feel you can be absolutely honest as you consider each of the questions. Just because you think something, doesn't mean you *have* to act on it. Get your thoughts down and then give yourself the time and space to decide if you want to make any changes or new choices.

Questions to Consider

- What effect is being a carer having on you, your health, your social life, your plans for your own life?
- What effect is being a carer having on your job or career?
- What impact is caring having on your income – can you afford to continue?
- How is your caring affecting other members of your family and your relationships with them?
- How is being a carer affecting your relationship with the person you're caring for?
- Is their condition getting any worse?
- Are they safe where they are with the current arrangements?
- How would you describe their quality of life?
- What changes might improve it? Why?
- How much longer do you think you will need to be a carer?
- Is it likely that the demands on you will increase?
- If they do, do you think you can cope?
- Do you feel you are coping now?
- What alternatives are available to you?
- Are you still the best person to be your loved one's prime carer?

CHAPTER 17

Moving to Residential Care

'In my experience, most people coming into a care home say they wish they had known what it was like in reality as they would have moved in sooner! Most care homes are good places to be. Unfortunately, the press is only interested in the horror stories so the perception is that all homes are terrible. They are not.'

Jill

Among the changes you may decide to consider once you've done your review is a move to residential care.

Let's all take a deep breath here. I'm well aware that for many of us that is the equivalent of a great big 'F' for Fail. We've all heard stories about how terrible these homes can be. And then, if you're caring for an adult, you've got their voice in your head telling you that the worst fate they can imagine is being 'shoved in a nursing home'.

Even if you're certain the time has come to consider residential care for the person you care for – and few carers are sufficiently detached from their own situation to see it quite so clearly – your resolve is likely to be clouded by feelings of sadness, loss and guilt.

Shouldn't you have been able to manage things better? Aren't you being selfish? Won't they be getting second-rate care if you're not there to deliver it? How awful would you feel if this was happening to you?

Your feelings are understandable – and familiar to all those carers who have ventured down this route before you. You may find it helps to share your feelings with someone who has personal experience of what you're now going through. A carers centre may be able to put you in touch or, when you start looking at residential homes, you can ask them for permission to contact the families of residents who are already in the home.

After a second stroke left Mum unable to move at all, my sister and I still hoped we could patch something together to continue caring for her at home. It took the compassionate support of Mum's adult social worker, the nurse in rehab, an occupational therapist, and two friends who'd been there and reluctantly gone down the care home route, to help us – and Mum – see we had done enough. Even so, Mum still had capacity and had she refused to go into residential care we couldn't have forced her.

Requesting a care review where you get input from such professionals who are bound to be more objective than you, see the bigger picture, and are trained to take both your loved one's and your best interests into account, may help you make the mental and emotional transition if, deep down, you know the time has come.

Seeing the possibilities in change

Remember, you have reached this point after looking at the impact of your caring role on everyone who is involved. What's in your best interests is almost certain to be in the best interests of others, too.

The other important thing to remember is that even if the person you care for goes into a nursing home, assisted accommodation or any other residential care setting, you haven't stopped being a carer – any more than your children leaving home means you're no longer a parent.

What it does mean is that you've got more time and energy for the best bits of a caring role – spending time with them, talking, sharing an activity, sharing memories or sharing feelings – while someone else is dealing with the day-to-day. Your loved one gets to meet more people and, hopefully, because you choose a good home, there'll be more activity and more interest in their days.

No one is asking you to stop caring about the quality of care the person you've looked after now gets. You'll be a point of liaison for whatever residential setting you choose, and any such setting worth its salt will positively welcome your involvement and your vast experience of caring for your loved one.

Choosing residential care

There is a whole range of things to consider when choosing a new care setting. And it's unlikely that you'll be able to cover everything in a single visit. Indeed, visiting any of the places you're considering at different times of day, with different staff on duty and other routines under way, will give you a more accurate picture of the quality and consistency of care each is offering. Talk to relatives of people already living in the home. When you visit, ask if there are any relatives around that you could speak to. Ask if there are any outside organisations that visit the home and make a note of them, then talk to them of their experience of the home.

Residential homes are reviewed by the same bodies who review care agencies in each part of the UK (see Chapter 14) so you can check the results of any recent inspection. But, frankly, this is an area where doing your own research, visiting, asking lots of questions, keeping your eyes open to even the smallest detail, asking around and talking to everyone you can, will serve you far better.

You can also ask for a trial stay first or arrange a period of respite that can be extended if the new arrangements are working well.

But let me just say that you might still get it wrong – and if you do, don't beat yourself up. Just do as you did as a carer and keep everything under review. If the home isn't as you imagined, or you can see things are no longer working there, then start the process all over again and find somewhere new.

What to look for and what to ask

It's almost impossible to do too much checking. So the suggestions below are only starters:

- How does the person you're caring for feel about the home?
- Do you like it? How would you feel about living there?
- Is it registered with a national or local association?
- What's the food like – can you both stay for a meal one day?
- Are visiting hours and numbers limited?
- Is it nicely decorated and is it clean?
- Does the home keep any pets or allow people to bring in their own?
- Can your loved one bring in their own items to make the space more personal?
- What does the daily timetable look like? What activities and services are available?
- How do the residents seem? Are they engaged and well cared for?
- How do staff talk to them?
- What proportion of residents are suffering from dementia? If your loved one is still mentally active, are there other residents they'll be able to talk to?

- How practical will it be for you and other family and friends to visit (distance, public transport routes, etc.)?
- How will the place be paid for? Can you afford it? If the council is picking up some of the bill, is there a top-up fee you'll still have to find?
- Can you get a clear breakdown of costs – some homes charge heavily for extras?
- Is there a recent inspection report you can see?
- Can the home put you in touch with the families of other residents for references?
- If your loved one's condition gets worse, do they have the facilities to keep them there – you don't want them to have to move again?
- How many of the staff are permanent and how many agency (which may mean lots of different faces all the time)?
- Does the home have a waiting list? If so, how long? Waiting lists are good and bad – a sign the home is excellent (but there's no point getting your hopes up).
- Can you see the contract in advance to understand what you're committing to?
- Can you have a trial run?

Paying for residential care

Unless your loved one is under eighteen or below the minimum savings threshold and doesn't own their own home, they'll almost certainly have to make a contribution towards the cost of residential care.

The rules on this are being reviewed constantly as the UK's social care budgets come under almost impossible strain. So I shall only give you the headlines here. For the latest position, check any of the carers organisation websites, consult Age UK, or the social work team at your local council. And do plan on seeking independent financial advice before you commit to anything.

If your loved one has almost no savings and owns no property – or they share their home with a partner or other family member who will go on living there – then it's likely their place in a care home will be partially or fully funded by the local council.

That's good news and bad – because what the council can pay is usually capped and not all residential homes are willing to accept a lower rate for rooms they'd normally let out at a much higher one. Some will require a top-up from your loved one (or you) to the full room rate.

There's another circumstance in which your loved one's place may be partially or fully funded and that's if they not only need care but also nursing. In that case, you or the home can request an NHS Continuing Care Assessment at which the local health commissioning body will work out what proportion of your loved one's needs come under the 'nursing' heading.

There's a full explanation of the assessment process on the NHS's own website https://www.nhs.uk/conditions/social-care-and-support/nhs-continuing-care/. If your loved one doesn't qualify for NHS continuing healthcare, they may still be eligible for NHS-funded nursing care, which is a flat rate contribution towards their nursing care.

Children and young people may receive a 'continuing care package' if they have needs arising from disability, accident or illness that can't be met by existing universal or specialist services alone.

Those circumstances aside, it will be down to your loved one to self-fund until their savings are depleted to the minimum threshold level. This is where the council's financial assessor reappears and wants to know all about your loved one's assets. Over and above a fairly modest sum they are allowed to keep, they'll be expected to fund their own residential care through any savings and, after those have gone, through the sale of their house.

It's definitely worth seeking independent financial advice on your loved one's options before all of these wheels start turning. There are particular circumstances, for instance, if their home is also occupied by someone else, where they may not be required to sell. And even if their home is decreed to be a part of their financial assets, an adviser will help you work through all options, such as borrowing the money for fees against the future sale of the house, including from the local council. Or renting it out – although few homes will come close to funding residential care fees which are terrifyingly high.

All of which said, there's no way of sweetening the fact that you've got to manage all this on top of everything else and, if your loved one's home does have to be sold, deal with their devastation at the loss of their home.

The best I can offer – having gone through the trauma myself – is that it's *their* money and always was. And what better way to spend it than on ensuring they have the best quality end of life that money can buy?

Continuing to care

You may not be able to make it perfectly all right for your loved one if they hate the idea of leaving their own home or yours. But choosing a setting where they can take the things that matter to them and where they retain a degree of autonomy will give you the best chance of the new arrangements working.

Bear in mind that neither of you should rush the decision. Finding the right setting and moving into it is a huge thing for you both and it may take months before life settles down enough for you to be able to judge whether the new arrangements are working. Hard as it may be, you need to hold your nerve until that point and be clear with your loved one that change is difficult for everyone and you both need time to get used to it.

In the meantime, make a point of getting to know those who have taken on the caring role as you would if they were coming into your home. You are still a part of a caring partnership and playing an active role in it will make it easier for you to spot any problems, raise any issues, and act as your loved one's advocate.

Letting go may be very hard for you. But it is a mistake to spend too much time with the person you care for in the early days thinking you can withdraw a little once they've settled in. Having you there all the time will slow the process of them adapting to their new situation and, believe me, you'll find it gets harder rather than easier to cut the time you spend there.

There are other ways of showing you care and are watching, apart from spending every minute of your spare time at their side. You can phone or drop them a note from time to time; everyone enjoys getting post.

And now's also a good time to enlist help from others. It may be easier for other relatives to visit because they no longer have to feel so guilty that you're the one carrying the load.

CHAPTER 18

Beyond Caring

'Did I get anything out of it? Yes, I think it made me appreciate the little things – trees, the sky, grass, colours – which a lot of people don't see because they have to go out to work to pay the mortgage and they have to work so hard. When I did get time away it was like seeing life through a different pair of eyes.'

Sarah

One in every two carers will be looking after their loved one for up to five years. Another 25 per cent of carers are involved in looking after someone for between five and ten years, while the final 25 per cent are carers for over ten years.

Whichever way you look at it, that's a big chunk out of anyone's life; long enough for different routines to have become ingrained, for your ideas and priorities to have changed. In short, for the world to look a very different place from the one you inhabited before you became a carer.

Many carers find the weeks, months and even years after their caring role ends as tough and emotional as what went before. They need help adjusting – and recognising there is something for them beyond caring.

An end to caring

Your caring role may end for a number of reasons – the person you've been looking after may die; you may be a young carer who is leaving the nest to go to college, take up a job, or start your own family; you may be a parent carer who's had to make arrangements for your child to be more independent by moving them into a supported living environment. Whatever the reason, be prepared for some fallout, and allow yourself time for coming to terms with what has happened.

You are facing more loss – which has been the theme of your life for a long time. However relieved you may be to be free of some of the day-to-day practicalities, you are facing the loss of a close relationship and the loss of a role which, even if you hated it, you were at least familiar with.

For some, like Janet, the loss of the parent she'd cared for ran deeper still. She told me, 'I was her rock, but I never realised how much she was my rock, too. So when she died, I was totally, totally lost. I knew I could go anywhere and do anything . . . but I didn't and I don't.'

After such an intense period pouring our energy into keeping someone else going, putting our own needs at the bottom of the pile, some of us lose sight of who we really are and how to go on with our lives; with the death of the person we cared for, or the end of our caring role, we realise we have lost our identity.

When the one you are caring for dies

For the remaining months of his life, we were totally at peace and comfortable together. No more self-consciousness. No unfinished business . . . In a way, this was my father's final

gift to me – the chance to see him as something more than my
father . . . the chance to see the common identity of spirit we
both shared.'

A carer's perspective from *How Can I Help?*
by Ram Dass and Paul Gorman

There are no rules about dying. The best any of us can hope for is a
'good death' and, as a carer, you will be doing your best to achieve that
for the person you care for, whether you are supporting them through
many years of slow decline, or a swift illness.

As part of that process, you may feel able to discuss with them their
dying, their wishes for the way they are cared for up to their death
and what they want to happen afterwards. You may even have had
the foresight to help them make a Living Will – also known as an
'advance directive' – in which they've had a chance to be clear about
what they want at the end of their life. Age UK has a useful factsheet
on advance decisions, advance statements and Living Wills if you
would like guidance on what's involved.

In other cases, you may sense that this is not something you'll be
able to discuss, or their condition may not allow you to do so. If so,
it's important that you find someone with whom you can share your
feelings, worries and practical concerns. Because your role brings
you so close to the one you're caring for, you are, to a great extent,
experiencing their dying with them. You need an outlet for all of the
difficult emotions that will bring up for you.

If you don't have friends or a partner to share what you're feeling
with, contact one of the excellent bereavement counselling
charities; you'll find their details in the resources section at the
back of this guide. Some carers centres run special programmes
for 'former carers'.

Those carers who have been able to talk about dying with the one they're caring for often find great comfort and relief in it. At a practical level, knowing what last services you can do for someone you've cared for feels like completing the circle. At an emotional level, your honesty at this time may bring you still closer, cementing what has been – for good or ill – one of life's most significant relationships for you both.

You may want to talk about how they wish to spend their last weeks, people they want to see, even places they may want to visit. If they're suffering from a terminal illness, you may want to discuss pain control and whether they wish to be revived should something happen. They may want to share what they are feeling with you, their fears, or that they are ready to die. You could discuss funeral arrangements, where they would like to be buried or have their ashes scattered.

Equally, there may be times when neither of you wants to talk, simply to share the silence together. Don't be scared of silence. You have been so busy for so long, that you may find it hard to sit quietly. But this really is a time when sharing peace is an important stage in the journey ending and beginning for you both.

Dealing with the practicalities of death

Once upon a time most people died at home and we all grew up knowing what to do. These days, we have less contact with death and its aftermath. The checklist below will help you know what steps you must take, but don't be afraid to ask your doctor or a funeral director if you're worried or unclear. Funeral directors in particular see an important part of their role as guiding people through the things that need to be done when someone dies:

1. *Call the doctor* – the doctor has to confirm the death and will write out a medical certificate giving the cause. If your loved one

dies in hospital, then one of the hospital's medical staff will
do this.

2. **Contact a funeral director** – if you have access to the Will or to its
   executors, then look at this before you contact a funeral director
   to ensure you're aware of any special wishes. You should also
   consult any relatives who may want a say in the arrangements.
   Then find a funeral director – personal recommendation is a
   good way to choose. The funeral director will take much of the
   load from you if you wish, guiding you through your choices,
   contacting the crematorium and/or the relevant people in
   whichever faith your loved one was part of – or a civil celebrant
   if you prefer. If you want them to, they'll arrange the floral
   tributes and place a notice in the paper. If you haven't already
   got a paid-up funeral plan, it's best to go into the funeral home
   with an idea of what you can afford to spend. Don't feel
   pressured into spending more than you want on expensive
   coffins and extras.

3. **Register the death** – you need to do this within five days of the
   death, ideally at the registrar's office within whose district
   your loved one died. If in doubt, contact your local council or
   library for details. You'll need to take the medical certificate of
   death that the doctor wrote, plus the following documents if
   you have them: your loved one's birth and marriage certificates;
   medical card; pension or benefit books; and proof of address. The
   registrar will want to know your loved one's full name (including
   maiden name, if appropriate), last address, date and place of
   birth, date and place of death, their occupation, details of any
   benefits they were receiving, including pension, if they were
   married, the name and occupation of their husband or wife and
   any previous marriage partners, and the name and date of birth
   of any marriage partner surviving them. You'll be given a death
   certificate, a certificate for burial or cremation and a certificate

of registration of death. See www.gov.uk/register-a-death for full information.

4. ***Arrange the funeral*** – the funeral can take place once you have given the certificate for burial or cremation to the funeral director. When it comes to the service itself, remember if you can that you are celebrating and commemorating a whole life rather than just the recent years of caring. Your loved one was not only a dependant, just as you are not only a carer.

5. ***Deal with the paperwork*** – you will need copies of the death certificate for when you contact any solicitors, banks and building societies and insurance companies to tie up loose ends. You should also contact the Benefits Agency to cancel a pension or any other allowances, and if no one is going to be living in their house now, contact the services such as gas, electricity, water, phone and broadband companies, and the local council about Council Tax. The Government online tool called Tell Us Once to notify all official agencies and council departments is also very useful – if it's available in your area, you could save a lot of time and effort by using this service. See the resources section for more details.

Riding the emotional roller-coaster

One of the effects of all this activity is to take your mind off both your loss and the future so don't be surprised if you don't feel the need to grieve straight away. Some carers feel guilty because they think they should be more upset. Others worry that because they feel fine, even relieved, they couldn't have loved the one they've just lost enough.

The same is true if the person you were caring for has moved into a new setting and is being cared for by others. There is a flurry of activity around making the new arrangements and winding up old ones, all of which postpones the moment when it is just you, and the silence, and the knowledge that your life is going to be different from now on. It's important you tell yourself that whatever you're feeling at this stage is very, very normal. You have been through a huge amount; your body and mind need time and space to process this before you begin to think about the future.

Loss and bereavement have their own patterns and timetables for each of us. It is normal to feel pain, sadness, anger and devastation; to experience denial – disbelief that anything has changed – and for your emotions to rise and fall randomly as if you were on some kind of unpredictable roller-coaster.

One of the first things you may experience is a sense of relief. Have you ever played that game where you stand in the doorway and push your arms out against the frame? When you stop, your arms fly up of their own accord, like wings. Ceasing to be a carer can feel like that. The pressure is off and the sense of light-headedness is intoxicating. And yet, after a few moments, your limbs fall back to your side, as heavy as ever. On the emotional roller-coaster, there's a down for every up; every positive feeling has its opposite. You need to go with all those emotions, allowing them to run their course, and using the following to guide you:

- Talk through the pain or confusion with those close to you as much as you need to. Expressing our feelings over and over again is our way of working through them.
- Be gentle with yourself. All the time you were a carer you were putting other people ahead of you. Now it really is time to take care of yourself.
- Don't be afraid of your emotions – they may be all over the place. You may be weeping one moment, angry another and laughing the next as you recall something funny from the past. Whatever you feel is OK.
- Get professional support – your local carers centre know that ceasing to be a carer is not like pressing a light switch onto 'off'.

That's why they will still classify you as a carer for twelve months after your role has ended. Talk to them and think about taking up any suggestions they make, whether that's seeing a counsellor for a few sessions or joining a support group. If that's hard for you, join one of the online forums for carers.

- Honour your memories. Hopefully, there were some good times as well as the challenging times and both are now part of who you are. Spend time with photo albums or souvenirs, allowing yourself to feel whatever emotions come up.

- Honour yourself – take the time to recognise, perhaps in a journal, why you were a carer, what you were able to give in that role and what you learned about yourself, other people and life through your contribution to someone else's well-being.

- If your loved one has died, buy a book on bereavement or contact one of the bereavement charities. There is great comfort in being reminded that death is something all of us experience and there are many people willing to understand what you are going through, share their experiences and show you that at some point you will come out the other side.

Be aware, however, that if the roller-coaster seems endless and shows no sign of slowing down, or you realise that no matter how much you talk the pain never seems to ease, you may need professional support. To grieve is normal; to be emotionally up and down for months, even several years, is also a familiar pattern to anyone who has experienced a major loss. But to find yourself incapacitated by grief means you need help – this is not your fault, simply a reflection of how deeply being a carer has affected you.

Facing up to the future

You may have given up a great deal to be a carer – your job, or at least your chances of a career, your friendships, relationships, hobbies, interests, holidays . . . the list goes on and on.

If so, the future may, for a while, look very scary indeed. So many minutes to fill, and you have very little idea of what to do with them. At first, you think how much you'll enjoy taking yourself off for a walk in the park or a coffee with friends but there's less pleasure in it than you'd expected. You're so used to being busy you can't adjust to having nowhere you need to be, nothing that desperately needs to be done.

Some carers experience a loss even deeper than the loss of their carer role. Having lived on the borders of someone else's life rather than at the centre of their own, they have lost the direction they once had and are left wondering what to do with their lives.

Consider how often, in social situations, you are asked, 'What do you do?' The society we inhabit has a way of pigeon-holing us according to the roles we fulfil. Retired people already know this; without their 'job', they are lumped together with everyone else over a certain age. If, for however many years, you have thought of yourself primarily as a carer, or that has been a significant part of 'what you do' – your identity – then like someone newly retired you may feel overwhelmed by the empty spaces, the choices and decisions that confront you, or that you know you need to take. That blank sheet can feel very scary indeed.

For others, the huge 'what next?' question mark hovering over their heads is simply pragmatism. If ten or twenty years have gone by since you started caring you may well no longer want the same things you did long ago. The world of work may have moved on and left you behind. Being a carer may have changed what you want out of life, and you simply haven't had time to think about putting any other dreams or ambitions in place of old ones that are now redundant.

Do think about getting help at this crucial time. All of a sudden, the social workers, care assistants, home helps and health professionals who offered you at least a little support have vanished from your life. But there are others able to step into the gap and ensure that you're cared for. You do have a future and you're owed help deciding what it will look like.

Keep this checklist close by and consult it often:

Care Plan for Former Carers

Do get support from friends, family, counsellors and carers support groups.

Do consult your doctor if you think you need medical help; for instance, if you feel exhausted all the time or depressed.

Do get lots of rest. However well you've managed, your batteries are in need of extended recharging.

Do make plans for difficult days if the person you cared for has died. Birthdays and anniversaries can be specially hard and you need to spend them with people who will understand your mixed emotions and be willing to listen. Or have permission from yourself to spend them alone.

Do get a health check – your health may have suffered or been neglected. It's time to focus on you.

Do expect to give yourself a decent period of 'time off'.

Don't allow others to rush you into things. They mean well but, for the first time in a long time, your time is your own.

Don't make any decisions about the future quickly. For a while, simply be open to any and every possibility until you are ready to make your own choices.

Don't let anyone tell you you must be glad it's all over. Your feelings are far more complex than that.

Don't worry if you suffer 'relapses'. Few of us live our emotional lives in a straight line.

Don't reproach yourself that you could have done more. You did the best you could at the time.

CHAPTER 19

Caring for the Carers

'Having been a paid carer myself, I know how hard I worked, how often I stayed late unpaid and how much I genuinely cared for patients, families and other colleagues. I also watched my mum as a community nurse for twenty-five years transform the lives of the dying and sick patients she looked after. I know not all paid carers were like me but my main frustration would be for the "system". It was so frustrating for us to be bogged down by paperwork when we wanted to spend time caring.'

Annie

This book is for and about carers. But as I was thinking about this new edition, I realised that one hope I have for it is that those people I've been calling 'the professionals' might find it helpful to know a little more of the challenges unpaid carers face – and how they could better support us.

Of course, it's tempting to say that the answer is 'more resources'. Life would be a whole lot better for all of us if there was simply more hard cash in the national and local budgets to fund better care, more support, more staff, more respite, and a carer's allowance that someone could actually live on. All of which is true, but since every national and local carers support organisation, and many other charities, have been saying this loudly for a very long time, I'm not sure it's going to get you and me very far to spend too many paragraphs on it.

If policymakers want to know why more resources would help, they only need to read this book or listen to any of the organisations that have been campaigning so hard and so long. For now, let's not try to move the whole mountain. Let's instead dig in with a few practical suggestions that will help the professionals take away just a little of our load.

As I do so, I want to give an honorable mention to those professionals who not only trained to do the jobs they do because they wanted to help people and make the world a fractionally kinder place, but continue to do those things in the face of endless red tape, massive workloads and unprecedented pressure on budgets.

Thank you for all you do.

And thank you for sharing with your colleagues these thoughts from carers.

Professionals – how to help us help you

- Give us information – I wrote this book because I didn't know anything and I didn't know what I didn't know. It's taken me years to understand what help *is* available, and I'm still learning.
- If you do nothing else, give us the details of carers support organisations *whether or not* you think we need support.
- Treat us as your equals – as you would other professionals. That includes a respect for our time, our other commitments and our knowledge.
- We want to be heard and taken seriously. There may be correct procedural ways to accomplish things but a lifetime of living

cheek by jowl with an individual gives us a unique perspective on how to oil the cogs.

- Please don't use the expression 'What you could do is ...'. We accept there are a million things we could be doing but we already feel we are doing hundreds of them. We don't need advice that results in more work for us.
- And on the subject of time, please *be* on time. Many of us move heaven and earth to get to appointments and when you're late we can't help feeling your time is somehow more important than ours.
- Remember that communication matters hugely. Even if you've got no news, call or email us to tell us that so we know we've not been forgotten. And if you've promised to get back to us, do so. Things that are just one item on your pages-long to-do list may be matters of life, death or at least sanity to us.
- Never assume we're OK. Always ask how we are doing in case we've stopped coping and haven't realised it yet.
- In fact, please start every conversation with us by asking, 'How are you?'

Supporting your family member who is a carer

For any relatives who happen to pick up this book, here are some more suggestions for ways in which you can help the carers in your life:

- Always start by asking us how *we* are, rather than about the person we're caring for.
- Then ask how you can help. It's OK to be honest about how much time you have available. Look at the ideas in the Help List in Chapter 15 for practical help and gently suggest which you could do.
- Think about the ways in which you could occasionally give us respite for an hour or two. Again, there are plenty of suggestions in this book. Time out is probably the thing we crave the most.

- Don't let us down unless it's a genuine emergency. If you've offered something at a particular time, we really need you to come through.
- Don't take our moods personally; they are almost never about you.
- Actually, just being a great listener would help us a lot at such times. Most listening is people waiting to say *their* bit. If you can stay quiet and really *hear* us, that would mean the world.
- Don't expect us to make the effort to stay in touch with you. We're not ignoring you – we're just mad busy and will appreciate you making the running with us while this continues.
- Recognise the contribution we're making to someone else's quality of life. Carers are so often invisible that just honouring what we do from time to time helps us remember why we're doing it.

Carers' tips for carers

I asked all the carers I interviewed: 'What's the single most important piece of advice you'd give to other carers?' Here's what they came up with:

- You may be in it for the long haul. Pace yourself and keep something back for you.
- Don't expect to be perfect.
- It's OK not to know what to do for the best sometimes.
- Sometimes you'll get it wrong. We all do.
- Join a carers support group.
- Use technology wherever you can – for shopping, prescriptions, etc. – so you can spend quality time with the person you're caring for.
- Whatever it takes, make sure you have some back-up so you can take time for you.
- Define your boundaries and then stick to them. Never carry on without a break in sight.

- Try to be patient and understand sometimes the things that are happening are not in your control and you can only do your best even though at times it may feel it's not good enough.
- Remember you are not a superhero.
- Try and find the funny side in things. Dark humour has literally saved my life on more than one occasion.
- It can get boring, and it's OK to admit that!
- Self-care is not the same as selfishness.
- It's definitely not all bad – the person you're caring for really does appreciate what you're doing even if they can't or won't show it.

RESOURCES

Many of the organisations that appear below have separate offices in England, Northern Ireland, Scotland and Wales. Some also have an extensive network of regional or local branches. To simplify this section for readers, I have, in most cases, given contact details for the organisation's headquarters, from whom you'll get up-to-date information on who to contact in your part of the UK.

On the whole, I have only included phone numbers where they offer practical helplines. Many organisations now insist on you filling out an online enquiry form rather than making it easy to phone them.

The list is not comprehensive because including everything would have meant writing a second book! However, I am always happy to hear suggestions from you, the readers, of other services you have found invaluable and would like to recommend to other carers.

National Carers Organisations

Carers Trust

A major charity providing a wealth of resources for, with and about carers, with independently-run network partners offering services locally.

https://carers.org
Head office: 0300 772 9600
Scotland office: 0300 772 7701
Wales office: 0292 009 0087

Carers UK

National membership charity for carers, operating as a support network and movement for change – as well as an excellent source of information and advice.

www.carersuk.org
Careline: 0808 808 7777
Carers UK: 020 7378 4999
Carers Wales: 029 2081 1370
Carers Scotland: 0141 445 3070
Carers Northern Ireland: 02890 439 843

Other Sources of Information, Advice and Helplines for Carers

Age Space

Online resources and community for anyone caring for an elderly parent, relative or friend.

www.agespace.org

Age UK

Information, advice and practical services and support from more than 150 local Age UK branches.

www.ageuk.org.uk
Tel: 0800 055 6112

British Red Cross

Support at home, transport, first-aid training and mobility aids to help people in their daily lives.

www.redcross.org.uk

Caregiver Warrior

There are many excellent blogs by carers out there. This is one of my favourites for its humanity and compassion.

www.caregiverwarrior.com

Carers Direct

NHS guide for people needing care and those caring for them.

www.nhs.uk/conditions/social-care-and-support
Carers Direct Helpline: 0300 123 1053

Carers World Radio

Online radio station debating carers' issues.

www.carersworldradio.com

Independent Age

Information and advice aimed at helping people retain their independence as long as possible, with a section for carers, too.

www.independentage.org
Helpline: 0800 319 6789

My Ageing Parent

Website with information, shop and forum aimed at helping people care for an ageing loved one.

https://myageingparent.com

Which? guide for carers

Resources include an advice tool and care services directory.

www.which.co.uk/elderly-care/for-carers

Support for Young Carers

Action for Children

www.actionforchildren.org.uk/what-we-do/children-young-people/supporting-young-carers/

Barnados

www.barnardos.org.uk/what_we_do/our_work/young_carers.htm

Carers Trust

https://carers.org/about-us/about-young-carers

Carers UK

https://www.carersuk.org/help-and-advice/practical-support/

Childline

www.childline.org.uk
Tel: 0800 1111

Children's Society

www.childrenssociety.org.uk/youngcarer/home

Useful Links to Government Services

Online gateway through to a range of links relevant to carers: www.gov.uk/browse/disabilities/carers

Attendance allowance: www.gov.uk/attendance-allowance

Benefits calculator (links to a number of benefits calculator services): www.gov.uk/benefits-calculators

Carer's allowance: www.gov.uk/carers-allowance

Carer's credit (national insurance credit if you care for more than 20 hours a week): www.gov.uk/carers-credit

Direct payments: www.gov.uk/apply-direct-payments

Personal Independence Payment (PIP – financial help for 16–64-year-olds with the extra costs caused by long-term illness or disability): www.gov.uk/pip

Financial help for disabled people (overview of and links to possible sources of financial help): www.gov.uk/financial-help-disabled

Help for people caring for a disabled child (gateway to range of financial and practical support services): www.gov.uk/help-for-disabled-child

Pensions (pension calculator, pension claims and protecting your pension): www.gov.uk/contact-pension-service

Pension and savings credit: www.gov.uk/pension-credit

Power of Attorney and acting for someone who lacks capacity: www.gov.uk/government/organisations/office-of-the-public-guardian

Sources of Advice on Money, Debt, Benefits, Health and Social Care, Rights and Legal Matters

Advice Now

Independent not-for-profit website run by the charity Law for Life.

www.advicenow.org.uk

Citizens Advice

Free, independent, confidential and impartial advice to everyone on their rights and responsibilities, via webchat, or by phone or face-to-face locally.

www.citizensadvice.org.uk

National Debtline

Free, impartial and confidential advice on dealing with debt.

www.nationaldebtline.org
Helpline: 0808 808 4000

PALS (Patient Advice and Liaison Service)

The Patient Advice and Liaison Service (PALS) offers confidential advice, support and information on health-related matters. They provide a point of contact for patients, their families and their carers in your local area. Contact them via your local hospital or surgery.

Pensions Advisory Service

Free and impartial guidance on workplace and personal pensions.

www.pensionsadvisoryservice.org.uk
Helpline: 0800 011 3797

SEAP (Support, Empower, Advocate, Promote)

Independent advocacy to help resolve issues around health and social care services.

www.seap.org.uk
Tel: 0330 440 9000

Turn2Us

Helping people in financial need access benefits, grants and support services, plus a benefits calculator tool.

www.turn2us.org.uk

Counselling Services

BACP (British Association for Counselling & Psychotherapy)

A trusted route to finding an accredited counsellor.

www.bacp.co.uk

Counselling Directory

Another directory allowing you to search for a counsellor near you.

www.counselling-directory.org.uk

Relate

Support with all types of relationship challenges through local centres.

www.relate.org.uk

Youth Access

Free and confidential counselling, advice and information for young people from members of the Youth Access network where you live.

www.youthaccess.org.uk

Grant-making and Practical Support Services

The contacts below are only a start. Some of the charities listed in this section offer small grants themselves or can assist in accessing the UK's many local, regional and national grant-making trusts.

Family Fund

Grant support for the families of disabled children, plus signposting to other support services.

www.familyfund.org.uk
Tel: 01904 550055

Royal British Legion

Financial, social and emotional support to service people, their dependents and carers, including grant-making, care and respite.

www.britishlegion.org.uk
Helpline: 0808 802 8080

SSAFA (the Armed Forces Charity, formerly known as the Soldiers, Sailors, Airmen and Families Association)

Financial and practical support for serving and former service people and their families.

www.ssafa.org.uk
Helpline: 0800 731 4880

Mental Health Organisations

Mind

Advice and support for anyone with a mental health issue, including how to cope as a carer.

www.mind.org.uk
Infoline: 0300 123 3393

Rethink Mental Illness

Advice, information, support groups and campaigning to support people living with mental illness.

www.rethink.org

Samaritans

24-hour access to a confidential place to turn for listening and conversation, especially in a crisis.

www.samaritans.org
Helpline: 116 123

SANE

Emotional support and information for anyone affected by mental health problems through a helpline and online support forum, plus campaigning on education and improving mental-health services.

www.sane.org.uk
SANE-line: 0300 304 7000

Young Minds

Advice for young people on a wide range of issues that can affect their mental health, plus helpline for parents.

https://youngminds.org.uk
Parents Helpline: 0808 802 5544

Work, Education and Training

ACE Education

Independent information and advice on concerns with State education in England and Wales to parents of 5–16-year-olds, including special educational needs.

www.ace-ed.org.uk
Advice line: 0300 0115 142

Employers for Carers

Resources for employers who want to be more carer-friendly – co-ordinated by Carers UK.

www.employersforcarers.org

Future Learn

Free online courses from top universities and specialist organisations.

www.futurelearn.com

Learn Direct

Portal to wide range of online skills, training and employment services.

www.learndirect.com

Listening Books

Postal and Internet audio book service.

www.listening-books.org.uk
Tel: 020 7407 9417

National Extension College

Wide range of courses available for home study, including GSCE, A-level, professional and personal interest programmes.

www.nec.ac.uk
Tel: 0800 389 2839

Open University

Distance learning courses, from short courses in creative writing and family history through to degree and postgraduate level study.

www.open.ac.uk
Tel: 0300 303 5303

U3A (University of the Third Age)

Bringing together people in their 'third age' to develop interests and continue informal learning through a network of local groups.

www.u3a.org.uk

Working Families

Helping working parents and carers and their employers find a better work-life balance, with a legal hotline for employment rights.

www.workingfamilies.org.uk
Advice line: 0300 012 0312

Home Care, Residential Care and Hospices

Care Inspectorate

Regulates and inspects care services in Scotland.

www.careinspectorate.com

Care Inspectorate Wales

Regulates and inspects care services in Wales.

https://careinspectorate.wales

Care Quality Commission

Regulates, inspects and rates care homes, home care agencies and mental health and community services in England.

www.cqc.org.uk

Hospice UK

Information on the work of hospices and hospice finder.

www.hospiceuk.org

Regulation and Quality Improvement Authority

Regulates and inspects care services in Northern Ireland.

https://www.rqia.org.uk

Relatives and Residents Association

Supporting residents, their families and carers to find out all they need to know about care and help when things go wrong.

www.relres.org
Helpline: 020 7359 8136

Sue Ryder

Hospice and care in the community, practical and emotional support for people facing a life-changing diagnosis, and those who care for them.

www.sueryder.org

United Kingdom Home Care Association

Advice on choosing care and searchable database of organisations providing care, including nursing and live-in care, to people in their own homes.

www.ukhca.co.uk
Tel: 020 8661 8188

Disability and Accessibility

See also the listings for charities representing specific disabilities in the general listings below.

Ability Net

Helping people of any age or disability to use technology in education, at work, or in the home.

www.abilitynet.org.uk
Tel: 0800 269 545

Contact

Charity offering advice and support to families with disabled children.

https://contact.org.uk
Helpline: 0808 808 3555

Dial UK

Disability information and advice through an advice line and network of local centres.

www.dialuk.info

Disability Rights

Information, advice and campaigning by disabled people for disabled people.

www.disabilityrightsuk.org

Disabled Living Foundation

Impartial advice, information and training on independent living.

www.dlf.org.uk
Helpline: 0300 999 0004

Motability

Car and scooter lease scheme for disabled people.

www.motability.co.uk

Holidays and Respite

Disabled Go

Online register of accessibility information on restaurants, entertainments, railways stations, universities and more.

www.disabledgo.com

Disabled Holidays

Accessibility specialist travel agent in the UK and abroad.

www.disabledholidays.com

Leonard Cheshire Foundation

Supporting disabled people at home and in residential care, through respite and day services, as well as employment and digital inclusion projects.

www.leonardcheshire.org

Open Britain

Gateway to information on accessible tourism in the UK.

www.openbritain.net

Revitalise

Respite holidays for disabled people and carers.

www.revitalise.org.uk
Tel: 0303 303 0145

Bereavement

Bereavement Advice Centre

Free helpline and web-based information service on dealing with the death of someone close.

https://bereavementadvice.org
Helpline: 0800 634 9494

Compassionate Friends

Support for families mourning the death of a child of any age.

www.tcf.org.uk
Helpline: 0345 123 2304

Cruse Bereavement Care

Support, information and advice for children, young people and adults when someone dies.

www.cruse.org.uk
Helpline: 0808 808 1677

Tell Us Once

Information from the Government on what to do when someone dies and the Tell Us Once service.

www.gov.uk/after-a-death/organisations-you-need-to-contact-and-tell-us-once

Winston's Wish

Specialist support for children dealing with bereavement, and those supporting them.

www.winstonswish.org
Helpline: 08088 020 021

Pets

The Cinammon Trust

Working to enable people to keep their pets when they have difficulties at home, plus fostering and long-term care if the owner goes into care or dies.

www.cinnamon.org.uk

Information and Support Groups for Specific Conditions

All of the organisations below offer information, resources and advice. Some also have helplines and chat rooms where you can connect with others experiencing specific conditions. Many have a network of local branches where you can meet others face to face. Once again, this list is not intended to be comprehensive but a starting point for accessing support.

Action on Hearing Loss

www.actiononhearingloss.org.uk
Information line: 0808 808 0123

ADDISS (National Attention Deficit Disorder Information and Support Services)

www.addiss.co.uk
Tel: 020 8952 2800

Alzheimer's Society

www.alzheimers.org.uk
Helpline: 0300 222 1122

Anorexia & Bulimia Care

www.anorexiabulimiacare.org.uk
Helpline: 03000 11 12 13

Arthritis Care

www.arthritiscare.org.uk
Helpline: 0808 800 4050

BEAT Eating Disorders

For those with eating disorders.

www.beateatingdisorders.org.uk
Helpline: 0808 801 0677
Youthline: 0808 801 0711

British Heart Foundation

www.bhf.org.uk
Helpline: 0300 330 3311

British Liver Trust

www.britishlivertrust.org.uk
Helpline: 0800 652 7330

Cancer Research UK

www.cancerresearchuk.org
Helpline: 0808 800 4040

Colostomy UK

www.colostomyuk.org
Helpline: 0800 328 4257

Continence Foundation

www.continence-foundation.org.uk

Cystic Fibrosis Trust

www.cysticfibrosis.org.uk
Helpline: 0300 373 1000/020 3795 2184

Dementia UK

www.dementiauk.org
Helpline: 0800 888 6678

Diabetes UK

www.diabetes.org.uk
Helpline: 0345 123 2399

Down's Syndrome Association

www.downs-syndrome.org.uk
Helpline: 0333 1212 300

Epilepsy Society

www.epilepsysociety.org.uk
Helpline: 01494 601 400

Headway

The charity for those with brain injury.

www.headway.org.uk
Helpline: 0808 800 2244

Hft

For those with a learning disability.

www.hft.org.uk

Leukaemia Care

www.leukaemiacare.org.uk
Helpline: 08088 010 444

Leukaemia UK

www.leukaemiauk.org.uk

Macmillan Cancer Support

www.macmillan.org.uk
Helpline: 0808 808 00 00

Marie Curie Cancer Care

www.mariecurie.org.uk
Supportline: 0800 090 2309

ME Association

www.meassociation.org.uk
Helpline: 0844 576 5326

Mencap

For those with a learning disability, autism, Down's Syndrome.

www.mencap.org.uk
Adviceline: 0808 808 1111

Motor Neurone Disease Association

www.mndassociation.org
Helpline: 0808 802 6262

MS (Multiple Sclerosis) Society

www.mssociety.org.uk
Helpline: 0808 800 8000

National Autistic Society

www.autism.org.uk
Helpline: 0808 800 4104

National Osteoporosis Society

https://nos.org.uk
Helpline: 0808 800 0035

Parkinson's UK

www.parkinsons.org.uk
Helpline: 0808 800 0303

RNIB (Royal National Institute of Blind People)

www.rnib.org.uk
Helpline: 0303 123 9999

Scope

Specialists in cerebral palsy but inclusive of all disability.

www.scope.org.uk
Helpline: 0808 800 3333

Sense

For those who are deaf-blind and have complex communication needs.

www.sense.org.uk

SIA (Spinal Injuries Association)

www.spinal.co.uk
Helpline: 0800 980 0501

Stroke Association

www.stroke.org.uk
Helpline: 0303 3033 100

Terrence Higgins Trust

For those with HIV.

www.tht.org.uk
Helpline: 0808 802 1221

Further Reading

There are a number of books I found very useful when thinking about how to tackle this guide, what to put in and what to leave out. They are listed below.

Codependent No More: How to Stop Controlling Others and Start Caring for Yourself, Melody Beattie (Hazelden, 1986)

The Caregiver's Essential Handbook, Sasha Carr, M.S. and Sandra Charon (McGraw Hill, 2003) – experienced caregivers share time-tested ideas and advice

How Can I Help? Emotional Support and Spiritual Inspiration for Those Who Care for Others, Ram Dass and Paul Gorman (Rider, 1985)

C, John Diamond (Vermilion, 1998)

The Carer's Handbook (British Red Cross), edited by Jemima Dunne (Dorling Kindersley, 1997)

Past Caring, Audrey Jenkinson (Polperro Heritage Press, 2004)

Loving What Is, Byron Katie (Ebury, 2008)

Out of Winter, Carol Lee (Hodder and Stoughton, 2014)

Hello and How Are You? A Guide for Carers by Carers (Macmillan Cancer Support)

A Caregiver's Survival Guide, Kay Marshall Strom (InterVarsity Press, Illinois, 2000)

The Selfish Pig's Guide to Caring, Hugh Marriott (Polperro Heritage Press, 2003)

The Story of My Father, Sue Miller (Bloomsbury, 2004)

The Directory of Grant Making Trusts, Ian Pembridge (Directory of Social Change, 2017)

Stand Up for Your Life, Cheryl Richardson (Free Press, 2003)

Take Time for Your Life, Cheryl Richardson (Bantam Books, 2000)

Caring for Parents in Later Life, Avril Rodway (*Which?* Consumer Guides, 1992)

Keeping Mum: Caring for Someone with Dementia, Marianne Talbot (Hay House, 2011)

The Caregiver's Little Guide to Survival: 7 Fail-Safe Tips for Caregivers, Suzanne White (2018)

Make the Most of Being a Carer, Ann Whitfield (Need2Know, 1996)

ACKNOWLEDGEMENTS

I am immensely grateful to all of those friends and colleagues who cast a kind and expert eye on the manuscript, and made many useful comments and suggestions. Thanks in particular to Yvonne Cook, Jill Holmes, Caroline Jarrett and Helga Stiborski, all of whom brought a wealth of experience and knowledge to helping me fine-tune this new edition.

Much of the earlier editions survives in this new book, so I must also thank those who mentored and advised me first time around: Jackie Ruane, Peter Tihanyi on behalf of what was then the Princess Royal Trust for Carers, and Harvey and Katy Brown of the Milton Keynes Carers Project, who were generous in sharing with me their experience of working with carers, and introduced me to many. Dawn Steel, then at the Open University, and Annette Eden, for Milton Keynes Welfare Rights, gave me invaluable help with the sections on work and benefits.

Many carers agreed to talk to me and I am grateful for both their interest, but especially their honesty in sharing often very difficult experiences and emotions. Those who were happy to be credited by name are as follows: Jane Alexander, Tony Baxter, Michele Brenton, Ros Buckle, Linda Camborne-Paynter, Davinder Chauhan, Janet Cooper, Teresa Davidson, Jenny Doran, Annie Frere, Martha Henderson, Shirley Jones, Carol Kenneally, Hazel Matthews, Mary

McCabe, Tom O'Brien, Shirley Paley, Devinder Panesar, Debbie Prime, Joyce Statham, Daphne Whitehouse, Teresa Williams, Mary Wootton and Ingrid Wrathall. Others appear anonymously: you know who you are – thank you.

To the many more millions of carers out there who I haven't spoken to, but whose lives I've tried to understand, thank you for all you do. As Carers UK puts it: 'Caring is such an important part of life. *It's simply part of being human.* Carers are holding families together, enabling loved ones to get the most out of life, making an enormous contribution to society and saving the economy billions of pounds.'

Finally, and with a full heart, I want to thank my family – my sister and soulmate Shushie, who has shared every step of the ten-year journey we've walked and often stumbled as carers for our mum. To Tom, Amy, Paul, Pud and Bob, thank you for supporting us, putting up with us when the going gets tough, and for helping in a myriad practical and emotional ways – including sharing your own experiences not only of living with a carer, but being carers yourself. I have written that it is love that, in the end, drives me as carer. It is my love for you and yours for me that drives me every moment of my life.

INDEX

Note: page numbers in **bold** refer to care-related organisation's contact details.

Ability Net **193**
acceptance 127, 128
accessibility advice 193–4
accidents 70–1
ACE Education **190**
Action for Children **184**
Action on Hearing Loss **197**
ADDISS (National Attention Deficit Disorder Information and Support Services) **197**
advance directives (Living Wills) 167
advice 146, 181–201
  accessibility advice 193–4
  benefits 16, 37–8
  bereavement 195–6
  see also Citizens Advice
Advice Now **186**
advocates 19
Age Space 6, 95, **182**
Age UK 14, 33, 44, **183**
  and benefits advice 16
  Bladder and Bowel Problems publication 79
  and day centres 134
  and keeping fit 82
  and Living Wills 167
  and lunch centres 135
  and paying for residential care 161
alarm systems, personal 63–4, 68–9, 71

Alzheimer's disease 85
Alzheimer's Society **197**
anger, feelings of 113–16
Anorexia & Bulimia Care **197**
anxiety 120–1
appointees 44
Armed Forces Charity (formerly Soldiers, Sailors, Airmen and Families Association) (SSAFA) 41, **188**
Arthritis Care **197**
arts and crafts 134
assertiveness 34, 98
assessments 9, 26–8
  and employment 55
  financial 11–12, 17, 23–4
  home care xv
  NHS Continuing Care Assessment 162
  young carer's needs 105–6
  see also Care Act (needs) assessments
Attendance Allowance 39, 50, 133, 139, **185**
audits, mental 16
'automatic pilot' 153–4

BACP (British Association for Counselling & Psychotherapy) 148, **187**

balance of care 127
bank accounts 43
Barclays bank 51
Barnados **184**
BBC (British Broadcasting
 Corporation) 7
BEAT Eating Disorders **197**
benefits 16, 50
 advice 16, 37–8
 and becoming an appointee 44
 benefits calculator **185**
 finding out what you are entitled
  to 37–40, **185**
 missing out on 9
 non-means tested 39
 and state pensions 50
 see also Attendance Allowance;
  Carer's Allowance; carer's
  credit; Personal Independence
  Payment
Benefits Agency 170
benevolent funds 40
bereavement 112–13, 171–2
 advice on 195–6
 benefits 40
 charities 167, 172
 see also death of a loved one
Bereavement Advice Centre **195**
Blue Badge scheme 77–8
body language 34, 35
boundary setting 71–2, 126–7, 179
breakdowns xvii, 123
 see also burnout
breaks, taking 81
British Association for Counselling
 & Psychotherapy (BACP) 148,
 187
British Broadcasting Corporation
 (BBC) 7
British Heart Foundation **197**
British Liver Trust **198**
British Red Cross 14, **183**
bulletin boards 69
burnout xvii, 111, 123

cabin fever 76
calendars 70
Cameron, Judith 48

campaigning 147–8
cancer xiii, xvi, 134
Cancer Research UK **198**
capacity 88
 lack of 185
 and lasting power of attorney 43,
  44
 and moving to residential care
  158
car tax 40
care
 balance of 127
 choosing to care 3–4, 5–6
 'continuing care packages' 162
 distance-based 63–6
 duration of 165
 the end of caring 165–75
 respite care 12, 135–7, 160, 178,
  194–5
 see also home-based care
Care Act (needs) assessments 17,
  18–21
 for children 21–2
 involving your loved ones in 20–1
 and paid care 132
care agencies
 'interviewing' 131–2
 paying for care from 132–3
care assistants 12
care environment adaptations 18,
  67–9, 70–1
care homes *see* residential care
Care Inspectorate 132, **191**
Care Inspectorate Wales **192**
care managers 11
care maze 8–16
care plans 11–12, 19
 costs 23
 and direct payments 24
 for former carers 174–5
 and paid care 132
 reviewing 20
 signing 20
Care Quality Commission 132,
  192
care reviews 153–6, 158
care teams 31–3, 139
Caregiver Warrior **183**

carer support 140–52
  and asking for help 141–5
  and bereavement 171–2, 173–4
  and carers centres 145–7
  and cleaners 140
  and counselling 148–9
  and family and friends 149–50, 155
  gateway to 9
  and Internet resources 147–8
  and mental audits 16
  and support groups 145–7
  and young carers 184
carers
  becoming a carer xiii–xiv, 1–7
  caring for 176–80
  crisis points 10, 123–9
  defining 2
  health for 73–84
  invisibility of 3
  sandwich 7, 100–1
  subsidising of government spending 49
  UK numbers of 1, 6–7
  see also assessments; paid carers; relationships, carer-recipient; self-care for carers; survival; young carers
Carer's Act 136
Carer's Allowance 37, 39, 50, **185**
carers centres 14, 131
  and benefits advice 38
  and Blue Badge help 77
  and carer support 145–7
  and children with special needs 95
  and dealing with feelings of loss 113
  and the death of a loved one 167
  and young carers 104–5
carer's credit **185**
Carer's Creed 122
Carers Direct **183**
Carers Equal Opportunities Act 2004 55
carer's plans 55
Carers Trust **182**, **184**
  carer definition 2

and carer statistics 2, 7, 48
carers centres of 14
and employment 54
'Key Facts about Carers' document 9
and money matters 48
and young carers 103, 104
Carers UK **182**, **184**
  carers centres of 14
  and money matters 48
  and sandwich carers 101
  'State of Caring' survey 2017 9, 73, 119
  and young carers 105
Carers World Radio **183**
caring for the carers 176–80
cars 52
case workers 11
Centre for Longitudinal Studies 101
change 153–6, 158–9
child rearing 7
Childline 105, **184**
children, how caring affects 99–100
children with special needs 1, 2, 62, 67
  advice for caring for 185
  assessments for 21–2
  and benefits 37
  and carer-recipient relationships 93–4
  and the end of the caring role 166
  and mental health problems 94
  and money matters 40, 48, 49
Children's Society **184**
choices 88, 98
  and care plans 24
  choosing to care 3–4, 5–6
  'good enough' 95
  for young carers 104
Cinnamon Trust, The **196**
Citizens Advice 14–15, 33, **186**
  and benefits advice 16, 38
  and Blue Badge help 77
  and dealing with other people's money 44
cleaners 140
  see also home helps
clothing 65, 68

co-dependence 123
Colostomy UK **198**
communication skills 92–3, 96
community psychiatric nurses 12
comparison websites 51–2
Compassionate Friends **195**
confidentiality 31
Contact **193**
contact details 66, 70
continence advisers 13
Continence Foundation **198**
continence nurses 79
'continuing care packages' 162
control
    fear of giving up 10
    feelings of a loss of 5
'copers' 27
coping
    signs someone is no longer
        coping 64–6
    strategies 151
Council Tax 39, 170
counselling 148–9
    bereavement counselling 167
    directory of services 187
    relationship counselling 90, 91–2
Counselling Directory **187**
credit cards 51
crisis points 10, 123–9
    see also health crises (of the
        cared for)
Cruse Bereavement Care **195**
'curse of the strong' 19, 109
Cystic Fibrosis Trust **198**

Dass, Ram, *How Can I Help?* 167
day centres xv, 12, 134–5
day-to-day tasks 18
death certificates 168–9
death of a loved one xv
    discussing 168
    and the end of the caring role 165,
        166–8
    and feelings 167, 170–2
    'good' deaths 167
    practicalities of 168–70
    registering deaths 169–70
    see also bereavement

deep vein thrombosis (DVT) 29
dementia 3, 85, 89–90, 112, 114, 153
Dementia UK **198**
denial 171
Department of Work and Pensions
    44
dependence 90
    see also co-dependence
depression 73, 111, 123, 124–5
despair 123, 124–5
Diabetes UK **198**
Dial UK **193**
diet 65, 73, 80, 81–2
dietary supplements 81
dieticians 13
direct debits 51
direct payments 24–5, **185**
Directory of Grant Making Trusts 41
disability advice 193–4
Disability Rights **194**
Disabled Go **194**
Disabled Holidays **194**
Disabled Living Centre 67
Disabled Living Foundation 67,
    194
distance learning 58–9, 84, 146
distance-based care 63–6
district nurses 12, 67, 74, 79
doctors 12, 16, 33, 74
    and day centre care 134
    and the death of a loved one
        168–9, 174
    and incontinence 79
    and respite care 137
    see also General Practitioners
Down's Syndrome 10
Down's Syndrome Association **198**
duration of care 165
DVT *see* deep vein thrombosis

early onset dementia 89–90
eating disorders 197
education
    advice on 190–1
    distance learning 58–9, 84, 146
emergency plans 70
empathy 146
Employers for Carers 56, **190**

employment issues 16, 53–60
  advice on 190–1
  flexible working practices 54,
    56–7
  and good employers 55–7
  and home/remote working 56
  leaving work 49, 57–9
  and legal help 54–5
  staying employable 58–9
  and taking leave 53, 55, 56, 57
  and the transferrable skills of
    caring 59–60
  and working part-time 49, 56, 57
end of caring 165–75
Enduring Power of Attorney (EPA)
  44
environmental adaptations 18,
  67–9, 70–1
Epilepsy Society **199**
Equality Act 2010 55
executors 45
eye contact 34

Facebook 119
falls 75, 154
families
  and carer support 137, 149–50
  family matters 95–9
  supporting family member carers
    178–9
Family Fund 40, **188**
family meetings 15, 98
feelings 108–22
  anger 113–16
  anxiety 120–1
  bottling-up 110–11
  and the death of a loved one 167,
    170–2
  despair 123, 124–5
  expressing 111–12
  'feeling' 111–12
  getting help with 122
  guilt 117–18
  loneliness 118–20
  of loss 112–13
  releasing 111–12, 115–16
  resentment 116–17
  see also survival

financial assessments 11–12, 17,
  23–4
financial issues see money issues
fire safety 71
first-aid courses 74
food 49, 65, 80–2, 138–9
food-related equipment 68
forums 67, 113, 119
Free Will Weeks 45
freezing food 81–2
friends 66, 137, 149–50
funeral directors 168–9, 170
funerals 169, 170
fury 113–16
Future Learn **190**
future, the 172–4

gateway to support 9
General Practitioners (GPs) 12, 30,
  37
Gorman, Paul, How Can I Help? 167
government services 11, 13–14, 185
  see also local government
    services
government spending, carer's
  subsidising of 49
grants 40, 41, 188
Guardian blogpost 48
guilt 95, 108, 117–18
  and asking for help 145
  and the death of a loved one 170
  and distance-based care 65
  and moving to residential care
    157–8, 164
  and taking time to keep fit 82

hairdressing 134
hand washing 75
Headway **199**
health for carers 73–84
  carrying out medical procedures
    74–5
  incontinence 78–9
  moving and handling procedures
    75–6
  self-care 80–4
health crises (of the cared for) 15
health and safety issues 70–1

health services 11, 12–13, 39
health visitors 76, 134
Healthcare Travel Costs Scheme (HTCS) 39
heart conditions 91
help, asking for 130–9, 141–5
    assessing how easy you find asking for help 141–4
    difficulties with 9–10, 41
    and family and friends 137
    and homes helps 138–9
    loved one's objections to 138
    and respite care 135–7
    and taking holidays 135–7
    with your feelings 122
    see also day centres; lunch clubs; paid care
Hft **199**
hobbies 66, 119–20
holidays 135–7, 155, 194–5
home helps 138–9
    see also cleaners
home-based care 61–72
    advice on 191–3
    creating a good environment for everyone 71–2
    and environmental adaptations 18, 67–9, 70–1
    and getting organised 69–70
    and home care assessments xv
    and safety issues 70–1
home-from hospital plans xv
home-from-hospital co-ordinators 13
homes helps 138–9
    see also cleaners
honesty 146
hope 146
hopelessness 124
Hospice UK **192**
hospices xv, 13, 134, 191–3
    day centres of 134
hospital 13, 168–9
    home-from hospital plans xv
    home-from-hospital co-ordinators 13
houses, forced sale of 163
housing benefit 39

HTCS see Healthcare Travel Costs Scheme
human connection, time spent on 4
humour 146, 180
hygiene
    and carrying out medical procedures 75
    personal hygiene 65

identity, loss of 166, 173
income support 39
incontinence 78–9
Independent Age **183**
information-giving 177
    organisations for 196–201
information-sharing 30, 32, 35
Internet resources 147–8
    see also forums
invisibility of carers 3

Katie, Byron 127
keys 66

lasting power of attorney (LPA) 43–4
    for health and welfare 16, 43
    for property and financial affairs 16, 43–4
Learn Direct **190**
leave, taking 53, 55, 56, 57
Lee, Carol 64–5
Leonard Cheshire Foundation **194**
'letting go' 164
Leukaemia Care **199**
Leukaemia UK **199**
Listening Books **190**
live-in-carers 137
Living Wills (advance directives) 167
local government services 11–12, 132
    and Care Act assessments 18
    and financial help with special equipment 40
    and residential care payments 162
London Underground 76
loneliness of caring 6–7, 118–20

loss 112–13, 118–19
  and the death of a loved one 173
  and the end of the caring role 166
love xvii–xix, 4, 6
low vision specialists 13
LPA *see* lasting power of attorney
lunch clubs 134–5

Macmillan Cancer Support 14, **199**
mail-order catalogues 46–7, 64
Marie Curie Cancer Care 14, **199**
Marriott, Hugh, *The Selfish Pig's
  Guide to Caring* xvii, 31, 91
Masons 41
massage 134
ME Association **200**
meals, help with 81, 138–9
meals-on-wheels 81
medical history 66
medical procedures, carrying out
  74–5
medication 64, 65, 69, 70
  different forms of 75
  keeping a clear record of 32
meditation 80
memory, music 89
Mencap 135, **200**
mental audits 16
'mental capacity' *see* capacity
Mental Capacity Act 2005 88
mental health nurses 12
mental health organisations 188–9
mental health problems 111, 145
  children's 94
Miller, Sue 85, 87, 89
Mind **188**
mind, nurturing your 83–4
mistakes 30
mobility 66, 76–8
money matters xiv–xv, 36–47, 154
  advice on 186–7
  asking for help with 41
  benefits advice 37–8
  and caring in your own home 62
  difficult conversations 46
  direct payments 24–5, **185**
  financial assessments 17, 23–4
  financial record keeping 52
  getting money savvy 50–1
  getting practicalities in order
    45–6
  and help with health care costs
    39
  impacts of caring on 23, 48–52
  and lasting power of attorney 16,
    43–4
  looking after someone else's
    money 42–4
  and making a Will 45, 46
  need to know checklist 66
  and over-spending 88
  and paying for care 36–7, 132–3,
    161–3
  and residential care 161–3
  savings thresholds 37, 162–3
  signs of not coping with 64, 65
  and spending controls 46–7, 51–2
  tips from carers 51–2
  useful links for 185
  see also benefits
Motability **194**
motivations for caring xvii–xix
Motor Neurone Disease
  Association **200**
moving and handling procedures
  75–6
MS (Multiple Sclerosis) Society
  200
music memories 89
My Ageing Parent **184**

National Attention Deficit Disorder
  Information and Support
  Services (ADDISS) **197**
National Autistic Society **200**
national carers organisations 182
  see also Carers Trust; Carers UK
National Debtline **186**
National Extension College **191**
National Insurance contributions
  50
National Osteoporosis Society **200**
Native American tradition 97
neighbours 66
NHS Continuing Care Assessment
  162

night lights 70
night sitting 12
numbers of carers 1, 6–7
nurses
    community psychiatric 12
    continence 79
    district 12, 67, 74, 79
    mental health 12
    practice 74
nursing homes *see* residential care

occupational therapy/therapists 13,
    40, 67, 76, 134, 158
Office of the Public Guardian 44
Open Britain **195**
Open College 59
Open University 58–9, **191**
    Managing my Money course 51
overnight bags 70

paid carers xv, 131, 136
    assessing the efficacy of 133–4
    and caring for the carers 177–8
    decision to use 91
    getting recommendations
        131–2
    homes helps 138–9
    live-in-carers 137
    paying for 132–3
    and personal care 79
    residential care 161–3
pain control 168
PALS (Patient Advice and Liaison
    Service) **186**
panic attacks 148
Parkinson's UK **200**
partners
    caring for 89–91
    feelings regarding caring for
        112–13, 118–19
    how caring affects 100
    and sex 91–2
passwords 66
pension credits 39, 185
pensions 58, 185
    and becoming an appointee 44
    impact of caring on 50
Pensions Advisory Service **186**

personal alarm systems 63–4, 68–9,
    71
personal care 79
personal hygiene 65
Personal Independence Payment
    (PIP) 39, **185**
perspective-taking 97–8
pets, advice on 196
physical exercise 73, 80, 82
physiotherapists 13
Power of Attorneys 16, 43–4, 46,
    185
practical aids/equipment *see*
    specialist equipment
practical support services 188
practice nurses 74
professionals
    working with 29–35
    see also specific professionals
public transport 76–7
pulmonary embolism 29

questions, asking 30

re-mortgaging 52
ready meals 81
record keeping 15, 35, 69
    financial 52
Red Cross 14, 74, **183**
registrars 169–70
Regulation and Quality
    Improvement Authority 132,
    192
Relate **187**
relationships, carer-recipient 62,
    85–102
    becoming a parent to your parent
        86–8
    and Care Act (needs)
        assessments 21
    and caring for partners 89–91
    and children who remain
        dependent 93–4
    and communication skills 92–3,
        96
    continuing to be child and parent
        87–9
    difficult 21

and family matters 95–9
how caring affects those closest
to home 99–100
open and honest 20–1
positive 101–2
and sandwich carers 100–1
and sex 91–2
see also partners
Relatives and Residents
Association **192**
resentment 116–17
residential care 8, 12, 136
advice on 191–3
choosing institutions 159–61
and continuing to care/carer's
role in 163–4
moving to 157–64
paying for 161–3
and taking holidays 136
trial periods 160
resources 176–7
Internet 147–8
respite care 12, 135–7, 160, 178,
194–5
responsibilities, assessing your 127
rest 81, 174
see also breaks, taking
Rethink Mental Illness **189**
retraining 58–9
reviews see care reviews
Revitalise **195**
Richardson, Cheryl
Stand Up for Your Life 151
Take Time for Your Life 151
rights, young carers' 105–7
RNIB (Royal National Institute of
Blind People) **201**
Royal British Legion **188**
rushing about 71

St John Ambulance 74
Samaritans 149, **189**
sandwich carers 7, 100–1
SANE **189**
savings accounts 43
savings credit 185
savings thresholds 37, 162–3
Scope **201**

SEAP (Support, Empower,
Advocate, Promote) **187**
self-care for carers xvi, xvii, 5, 63,
80–4
and assessing the balance of care
127
extreme 151–2
lack of 10
and nurturing activities 151–2
see also carer support
self-kindness 129
Sense **201**
Serenity Prayer 127
services
and asking for help 10
for children with special needs
22
directory 185
paying for 36–7
understanding who does what 11
voluntary 11, 14–16
see also government services;
local government services; paid
carers
sex 91–2
shopping, food 49
SIA (Spinal Injuries Association)
201
slowing down 71
snacks 80, 81
social workers 11, 158
and assessment for children with
special needs 22
and Care Act assessments 18, 19
changing your 33
and paying for residential care
162
and respite care 136–7
socialising 66
solicitors 45, 46
specialist equipment 18, 67–9
costs of 49
financial help with 40
mobility 76
moving and handling procedures
76
second-hand 67–8
for staying safe 70–1

speech therapists 13
spending
    controls 46–7, 51–2
    over-spending 88
Spinal Injuries Association (SIA)
    201
SSAFA (the Armed Forces
    Charity, formerly Soldiers,
    Sailors, Airmen and Families
    Association) 41, **188**
stress 4, 73, 82
    and changing the way you think
        about things 128
    overload 148
    recognition 125
stroke xvi–xvii, 29, 46–7, 64, 88, 102,
    158
Stroke Association **201**
Sue Ryder **192**
suffering 114
suicidal thoughts 94
support *see* carer support; caring for
    the carers
Support, Empower, Advocate,
    Promote (SEAP) **187**
support groups 15–16, 67, 109, 119,
    145–7, 179, 196–201
survival 123–9
    and boundary setting 126–7
    and changing your patterns of
        thinking 128–9
    and depression 123, 124–5
    and despair 123, 124–5
    and stress 127

tai chi 82
Talbot, Marianne, *Keeping Mum:
    Caring for Someone with
    Dementia* 3, 114, 153
tax credits 39
teamwork 31–3, 139
telehealth 68–9
Tell Us Once online tool 170, **196**
Terence Higgins Trust **201**
'third-party mandates' 43
thought patterns, changing your
    128–9

time, feeling short of 9, 128
training
    advice on 190–1
    distance learning 58–9, 84, 146
trip hazards 70
Turn2Us **187**
TV licences 40

U3A (University of the Third Age)
    191
United Kingdom Homecare
    Association 132, **193**

values 5–6
VAT exemption 69
voluntary services 11, 14–16
    see also specific organisations

walking sticks/frames 76
wandering 85
wheelchairs 76–7, 154
Which? guide for carers **184**
White, Susanne, *The Caregiver's
    Little Guide to Survival: 7 Fail-
    Safe Tips for Caregivers* 130,
    140
Wills 45, 46, 169
    see also Living Wills (advance
        directives)
Winston's Wish **196**
work *see* employment issues
Working Families **191**
worry 120–1

yoga 82
YouGov 7
young carers 7, 103–7
    and carers centres 104–5
    charter for 106–7
    and the end of the caring role 166
    and needs assessment 105–6
    rights of 105–7
    support for 184
Young Minds **189**
Youth Access **187**